TEXTBOOK OF FOOD AND NUTRITION

Published by :
Lotus Press Publishers & Distributors

TEXTBOOK OF FOOD AND NUTRITION

Meenu Grover
M.A., Ph.D (Food Science)
Punjab University

Lotus PRESS
4735/22, Prakash Deep Building
Ansari Road, Darya Ganj,
New Delhi - 110002

Lotus Press : Publishers & Distributors
Unit No. 220, 2nd Floor, 4735/22, Prakash Deep Building,
Ansari Road, Darya Ganj, New Delhi- 110002
Ph.: 41325510, 98118-38000
• E-mail : lotuspress1984@gmail.com
www.lotuspress.co.in

Textbook of Food and Nutrition

ISBN : 978-81-8382-036-3

Printed & Published by: **Lotus Press Publishers & Distributors,** New Delhi-02

PREFACE

Food is any substance consumed by living organisms, including liquid drinks. It is the main source of energy and of nutrition for animals, and is usually of animal or plant origin. Nutrition is the way our bodies take in and use food. Foods that are great sources of nutrition are called nutrients. There are six different types of nutrients carbohydrates, fats, proteins, vitamins, minerals and water. Nutrients give us energy, growth, help repair body tissues, and regulate body functions. Therefore each nutrient can be vital to our health. Absence of adequate nutrients can cause certain diseases to take hold that can potentially result in death.

This textbook is a comprehensive cross section of the world's current literature on food and nutrition. It will help us fill in the blanks by supplying us with important information about eating healthier and controlling our diet intakes and nutrition. It also provides an excellent presentation of the basics of nutrition as well as practical tips to improve health. It will be an invaluable addition to the libraries of food service professionals, students of the culinary arts, and professional and amateur chefs everywhere.

Editor

CONTENTS

1

INTRODUCTION

Nutrition begins with food. The science of nutrition concerns everything that the body does with food in order to live, function, grow, and heal. Foods that are eaten on a regular basis make up a diet. Although geographic location and family traditions play major parts in forming dietary habits, food choices vary from person to person.

To a high degree, what people eat affects their health and their enjoyment of life. In turn, healthy habits and a happy outlook can improve the ways in which the human body makes use of food. With the help of the sun, plants make their food from chemicals in the earth, water, and air. Animals—human beings included—cannot make their own food but must eat plants, other animals, or both.

In the early 1990s the long-standing, traditional basic four food groups, consisting of meat, dairy products, grains, and fruits and vegetables, were reworked into the more balanced and healthy food guide pyramid. This pyramid has as its base the grain group; on the second level are the fruit and vegetable groups; on the third level are the meat and dairy groups; and at the top is the fats, oils, and sweets group.

FOOD PYRAMID

Grain Group

At the base of the food guide pyramid are breads, cereals, rice, pasta, and other foods made from grain. Human beings need more daily servings of these foods than any others because grain-based foods provide B vitamins, iron, carbohydrates, and some protein. Six or more daily servings are recommended. A serving, for example, is one slice of bread, one ounce (28 grams) of dry cereal, or one half cup of cooked pasta.

Fruit and Vegetable Group

The sources of most vitamins and minerals belong to these two groups. They also provide fiber, which contains no nutrients but aids in moving food through the digestive system. Three to five servings of vegetables and two to four servings of fruits should be eaten every day. One half cup of any fruit or vegetable counts as one serving.

Dairy and Meat Group

On this level are two groups of foods, such as milk, cheese, poultry, fish, and eggs, that come mostly from animals; notable exceptions are nuts and dried beans. These groups are quite high in protein, calcium, iron, phosphorus, the B vitamins, and zinc. Two to three servings from each group are recommended daily. Eight ounces (227 grams) of milk or 3 ounces (85 grams) of meat, for example, count as a serving.

Fats, Oils, and Sweets Group

The top of the pyramid includes foods that may add pleasure to eating but provide only calories and little nutritional benefit to one's diet. These foods include salad dressings, cream, butter, margarine, sugars, soft drinks, and candies. They should be eaten only sparingly. The American Heart Association recommends that no more than 30 percent of one's daily calories be derived from fat.

NUTRIENTS

To function, the human body must have nutrients. The nutrients known to be essential for human beings are proteins, carbohydrates, fats and oils, minerals, vitamins, and water.

Proteins

Proteins are made of amino acids, small units necessary for growth and tissue repair. Protein is the body's most plentiful substance except for water and, possibly, fat. Animal foods such as meat, fish, poultry, milk, and eggs are rich in protein. Good plant sources of protein are beans, peas, nuts, bread, and cereals. Combining plant sources, such as peanut butter with whole-grain bread or rice with beans, provides excellent protein. So does combining plant and animal sources such as cereal and milk or macaroni and cheese.

Carbohydrates

Starches and sugars are carbohydrates, the main source of the body's energy. Carbohydrates account for about half of the calorie intake for most Americans and up to four fifths of the calories in diets of African and Asian peoples. Carbohydrate-rich foods are also the main sources of protein for most of the world. Rice, wheat, corn, and potatoes are common rich sources of carbohydrates. Sugars are not essential foods. They provide energy (calories) but no nutrients. For that reason sugar is called an "empty calorie" food. Occasional sweets are not harmful to a healthy, active person, but excessive sugar can lead to tooth decay when eaten between meals, especially in sticky snack foods that cling to the teeth.

Fats and Oils

Fats and oils (which are liquid fats) are a concentrated source of energy. Fats in the diet are necessary for good health. They make certain vitamins available for use in the body, they cushion vital organs, they make up part of all body cells, and they help to maintain body temperature. Fats also delay pangs of hunger because a food mixture containing fat remains longer in the stomach. Nutritionists distinguish between different types of dietary fats, or fats in food. Saturated fats usually are solid in form and of animal origin.

In many typical diets, meat fat is the main source. It is known that saturated fats can raise the level of cholesterol in the blood. Cholesterol is a natural waxy substance made by the body. It helps to form digestive juices and does other important work. It is present in the body no matter what is eaten. When the body cells cannot absorb any more cholesterol, any excess begins to accumulate in the walls of the blood vessels and gradually narrows them. This condition may lead to a heart attack or stroke.

Minerals

Minerals are neither animal nor vegetable; they are inorganic. Almost all foods contribute to a varied intake of essential minerals. Most minerals are easy to obtain in quantities required by the body. A major exception is iron for children under age 4 and adolescent girls and women in the childbearing years. These groups need more iron than a normal diet may provide. Iron helps to build red blood cells. It also helps the blood carry oxygen from the lungs to each body cell. Rich sources of iron are meat, especially liver; egg yolks; and dark green vegetables.

Everyone at every age needs calcium. This mineral builds bones and teeth, and it is necessary for blood clotting. The best sources are milk and hard cheese. Others are leafy greens, nuts, and small fishes—such as sardines—with bones that can be eaten. Phosphorus works with calcium to make strong bones and teeth. A diet that furnishes enough protein and calcium also provides enough phosphorus. Other important minerals are sodium, potassium, iodine, magnesium, zinc, and copper.

Vitamins

The discovery of vitamins began early in the 20th century. It is likely that some still are undiscovered. Eating a wide variety of foods ensures getting enough vitamins whether or not they are identified. All living things need vitamins for growth and health. The body either cannot manufacture them at all or cannot normally manufacture them in sufficient amounts, and so must absorb them from food. Each vitamin has specific roles to play. Many reactions in the body require several vitamins, and the lack or excess of any one can interfere with the function of another.

Fat-soluble vitamins: Four vitamins—A, D, E, and K—are known as the fat-soluble vitamins. They are digested and absorbed with the help of fats that are in the diet.

Vitamin A is needed for strong bones, good vision, and healthy skin. It is found both in dark green and yellow fruits and vegetables.

Vitamin D is essential for children because it helps calcium and phosphorus to form straight, strong bones and teeth. With direct sunlight on the skin, the body can manufacture its own vitamin D. Infants and young children often need a vitamin D supplement. Vitamin D is added routinely to most milk during processing.

Vitamin D is already known to be vital for bone health. However, a recent study suggested that it may be more useful than calcium in protecting older women from factures associated with osteoporosis. Researchers assessed relations between postmenopausal hip fracture risk and calcium, vitamin D, and milk consumption.

Women consuming 12.5 μg or more of vitamin D per day from food plus supplements had a 37% lower risk of hip fracture than did women consuming less than 3.5 μg/day. In addition, the risk of hip fracture was not influenced by the amount of calcium intake from milk or supplements in these women. The researchers concluded that "Because women commonly consume less than the recommended intake of vitamin D, supplement use or dark fish consumption may be prudent."

Vitamin E helps to protect vitamin A and red blood cells. It is found in a wide variety of foods, and almost everyone gets enough.

Vitamin K is one vitamin that is made within the human body—by bacteria that live in the intestinal tract. Small amounts are found as well in the green leaves of spinach, kale, cabbage, and cauliflower and also in pork liver.

Women with a low vitamin K intake may be at increased risk of bone fractures. The researchers studied self-reported dietary vitamin K intake and measured bone mineral density (BMD) of the hip and spine in more than 1,100 men and almost 1,500 women 29-86 years old. Dietary and supplemental intakes of vitamin K were assessed with the use of a food-frequency questionnaire. The researchers also accounted for such factors as age, body mass index, smoking status, alcohol use, physical activity score, and menopause status and current estrogen use among the women. Women with the lowest vitamin K intake had significantly lower mean BMD than those with the highest intake of vitamin K. These associations remained after controlling for variables and after stratification by age or supplement use. However, no significant association was found between dietary vitamin-K intake and BMD in men.

Fat-soluble vitamins can be stored in the body for long periods. They are stored mostly in the fatty tissue and in the liver.

Water-soluble vitamins: The vitamin B group of several vitamins helps to maintain healthy skin and a well-functioning nervous system. B vitamins also help to convert carbohydrates into energy. Vitamin C, or ascorbic acid, is needed for building the connective tissue that holds body cells together. Vitamin C is essential for healthy teeth, gums, and blood vessels. It also helps the body to absorb iron. These water-soluble vitamins are not stored in the body for long. Good sources should be eaten every day.

Vitamin C is known to play an important role in the structure of the collagen composed membrane. Supplementing pregnant women's diets with vitamin C would prevent levels from the nutrient in white blood cells, where it is stored, from dropping.

For the study, 52 women in their fifth month of pregnancy were given either a placebo or 100 mg. of vitamin C each day for three months. As is typical during normal pregnancy, vitamin C levels in blood plasma decreased for all the women. However, the white blood cell concentration of the vitamin decreased only among women given the placebo.

Additionally, women who took vitamin C supplements experienced an increase in their white blood cell concentration of the vitamin. At delivery, less than 5%

of the women who received vitamin C supplements experienced premature membrane rupture, in comparison to nearly 25% of women taking the placebo. The researchers concluded that vitamin C supplementation maintains stores of the nutrient in white blood cells and "may have value in preventing premature rupture."

Commenting on the study, one researcher said it "contributes another piece of evidence that vitamin C is important in the events that lead to premature rupture of the membranes." More studies with ample power to detect a difference are needed to confirm the role of vitamin C in preventing premature rupture,". Extra vitamin C should not just come in the form of pills. Pregnant women should also be sure to eat lots of vitamin C-containing fruits and vegetables, such as citrus fruits and broccoli.

Water

In order to live, every cell in the body must be bathed in water. Water takes an active part in many chemical reactions and is needed to carry other nutrients, to regulate body temperature, and to help eliminate wastes. Water makes up about 60 percent of an adult's body weight. Requirements for water are met in many ways. Most fruits are more than 90 percent water.

CALORIES

The body's most basic need is energy. To get energy it needs food as a fuel and oxygen to burn it. The amount of energy foods can produce is measured in units called calories. A food calorie, or kilocalorie, is the amount of heat required to raise the temperature of 1 kilogram (2.2 pounds) of water 1 degree Celsius (1.8 degrees Fahrenheit).

The body changes the calories in food into energy,

which is necessary for every act from blinking an eye to running a race. Energy is also used for the growing process, for rebuilding damaged cells, and for regulating body systems. The number of calories needed each day depends upon how much energy an individual's body uses. An active child can need more calories than an adult who works at a desk. The body needs more calories in cold weather to stay at an even temperature.

If a person takes in more food than required to meet the body's needs, the excess calories are converted to fat—a stored form of energy. That causes weight gain. Eating too little causes weight loss because the fat is used for energy. One pound (0.5 kilogram) of stored fat contains about 3,500 calories. If weight loss is advisable, the best way to lose is by eating less of high-calorie foods and getting more exercise.

For most people a safe limit for losing weight is 2 pounds a week. Strict dieting to lose weight should be attempted only under a physician's care. So-called quick and easy weight-loss diets are fads. Most are unbalanced, emphasising one type of food and excluding others. The more unbalanced the diet, the more dangerous it is. Knowledge of the body's nutritional needs helps to guard against promoters of fad diets and special "health" foods that have no advantages and that may even be harmful.

2

FOOD AND NUTRITION TECHNOLOGY

Food safety as well as the health benefits from food pervading discussions in every sphere of society have become real, pressing concerns for consumers as they wonder whether the sources and objects of their dining pleasures are fraught with dangers to warrant their fear or constant vigilance.

Deficiency of Vitamin-A

More than 250 million children less than five-years old are exposed to the risk of vitamin-A deficiency worldwide. About 500,000 of them go blind annually and 2 million die from this deficiency every year (2003-2004). To address this deficiency, several strategies can be adopted: medical supplementation, i.e., prescribing vitamin-A pills; the enrichment of food with vitamin A in the agro-industry or when preparing food at the communitary level; and inducing the diversification of food resources that are locally available.

The latter strategy was adopted in a pilot project carried out in Burkina Faso, West Africa, in conjunction with promoting the consumption of non-refined red palm oil. From 1999 to 2001, in collaboration with researchers from the University of Montreal Department of Nutrition and from the Health Research Institute at Ouagadougou, Burkina Faso, scientists of the French Development Research Institute (IRD) Unit on Nutrition, Food and Societies, have tested the efficacy of red palm oil on the body's vitamin A as it tested these on mothers and children under five years of age in the centre-east of the country, where this oil is not usually consumed. This oil, well known for its high content of beta-carotene – a precursor of vitamin A – is produced and mostly consumed in the north-west of Burkina Faso.

Palm oil has therefore been transported to, and sold on, the sites of the pilot project in order to evaluate its impact on vitamin A deficiency under conditions where women bought the oil freely and voluntarily. The women were previously informed about the beneficial effects of red palm oil through debates, lectures, theatre performances, etc.. The impact of palm oil was evaluated among women and children, at the beginning and the end of the pilot project through testing the amount of retinol in the blood serum. Results showed that after two years, the quantity of vitamin A ingested by the mothers and children who consumed red palm oil increased markedly: increase from 41 per cent to 120 per cent of safety inputs among the mothers and from 36 per cent to 97 per cent among the children.

Simultaneously, the proportion of mothers and children having a retinol content in the serum lower than the recommended threshold (0,70 μmol/l) at the beginning of the study, has decreased from 62 per cent to 30 per cent for the women and from 84.5 per cent to 67 per cent for the children. These results demonstrated that red palm oil was an efficient food supplement in real commercial conditions for combating vitamin A deficiency. In addition, about half of the women involved in the study modified their eating habits within two years while voluntarily consuming this foodstuff that was new to them.

The consumption of red palm oil could therefore be incorporated, like other food items rich in pro-vitamin A (fruits and vegetables), into national programmes for controlling vitamin A deficiency in Burkina Faso, where the afore-mentioned pilot project is being extended, and in other countries in the Sahelian zone.

Artificial Sweeteners

Sucralose is an artificial sweetener that is arguably the food industry's hottest new ingredient, turning up in everything from the recently launched 'mid-calorie' versions of Coke and Pepsi, to low-carbohydrate ice cream. Yet this sweetener was actually invented in the 1970s. Its success has been the reward for the decades of toil by Tate & Lyle, the British ingredient-maker that patented the substance in 1976 and is currently selling it as a sugar substitute to food manufacturers. Johnson & Johnson, the US health-care group, is selling sucralose for home use under the brand name Splenda.

The innovative sweetener is actually chlorinated cane sugar (sucrose). During the manufacturing process, three hydrogen-oxygen groups on a sucrose molecule are replaced by three tightly bound chlorine atoms. The resulting molecule (sucralose) is about 600 times sweeter than sugar and passes through the body without being broken down. The chlorinated agent is sodium chloride, and the underlying chemistry has not put off consumers or food manufacturers. Tate & Lyle has calculated that the worldwide market for 'intense sweeteners' was worth $1- billion a year at manufacturers' selling prices.

In the relatively short time it has been available,

sucralose has picked up 13 per cent of this market, giving it second place behind aspartame's 55 per cent, according to Tate & Lyle. Its compatibility with low carbohydrate dieting, not to mention direct praise from the late Dr. Atkins himself, has helped. In the US, Splenda is now the leading sugar substitute, having surged ahead of the likes of Equal and Sweet'N Low. IRI, the Chicago-based market research company, revealed that Splenda accounted for 43 per cent of the sugar substitutes bought through US stores – excluding Wal-Mart – to May 2004. Sucralose is also making significant in-roads into the food-ingredients market.

Both The Coca-Cola Co. and Pepsi Co., Inc., were using it in their new 'midcalorie' colas, Coca-Cola C_2 and Pepsi Edge, which have been designed to contain half the calories of the regular offering without diluting the sweetness as much as current diet versions. Because it performs better at staying sweet at high temperatures than other artificial sweeteners, sucralose can be used in foodstuffs that previously relied on sugar, such as microwaveable popcorn. Because of its better sweetening performance at high temperatures, McNeil Nutritionals, the Johnson & Johnson's unit responsible for Splenda, was persuaded to introduce a bigger pack size for Splenda to cater for demand from bakeries. This 5lb 'baker's-bag' retailed at Rs. 315-360.

Although the original patent dated back to 1976, sucralose had to wait until the 1990s for the first wave of regulatory approvals to come through. In 1991, it was cleared by Canadian authorities. Australia gave it the go-ahead in 1993. Tate & Lyle applied for US approval in 1987. After a long time preparing all the technical information required for the application, US clearance was granted in 1998. In the EU, sucralose had already been available in the United Kingdom, Ireland and the Netherlands but only gained approval for use in all

European countries by early 2004 after the publication of an amendment to the EU sweeteners directive.

The swelling demand for sucralose led to speculation that the sole manufacturing plant in McIntosh, Alabama, might not cope. The factory used to be jointly owned by Tate & Lyle and McNeil Nutritionals, but the British company took full ownership in 2004 as they redrew their sucralose partnership. In June 2004, Tate & Lyle announced the plant would be expanded at a cost of Rs. 1450, the work being completed in January 2006. As for its safety to consumers' health, sucralose has faced claims spread through the Internet, as aspartame had been in its time, that it was not safe, in spite of obtaining official clearance in many countries. However, the Center for Science in the Public Interest, a US lobby group noted for its scepticism of the food industry, declared that there was no reason to suggest that sucralose caused any harm.

HEALTHIER FOOD PRODUCTION

Our eating habits have changed dramatically during the 20th century. In the first 50 years, especially in the immediate aftermath of World War II, food was simply a source of energy. Today it is also a sensory, cultural and social phenomenon. As well as providing enjoyment, we now want food to enhance our health and well being. Furthermore, many of us are no longer willing to spend scarce leisure time preparing elaborate meals. Our food has to be quick and convenient to prepare, as well as healthy and tasty. Finally, we expect our food to be reasonably priced.

We may take all this for granted, but catering to a market of more than 350 million people in central Europe alone is no easy task. Moreover, as the population grows, the number of agricultural growers is declining. This increases the pressure on transport and storage systems, especially since many raw materials are not grown in

Europe. It may seem impossible to meet all the demands. However, technological progress in food manufacturing and recent discoveries in nutritional science have resulted in increasingly high food quality standards and enormous food variety.

Many of us could improve the imbalance between calorie intake and physical activity. However, in recent years there is evidence that recent discoveries about diet are starting to have an impact on our eating habits. We are now more inclined to choose lean meat, vegetables, and foodstuffs high in dietary fibres.

As modern nutritional sciences provide more information about the mechanisms by which certain food ingredients influence our body functions, scientists and market experts agree that foods with a declared positive impact on health are growing in popularity. Market analyses of consumer demands and behaviours forecast that within the next few years, nearly every product group will include special health-enhancing foods. Science focuses on reducing risk for chronic illnesses and debilitating diseases, particularly on cardiovascular diseases, obesity, cancer, osteoporosis and non-insulin dependent diabetes.

Today, consumers expect convenience food to be quick and easy to prepare and to meet high nutritional standards. Although there are some niches left where it is not possible to buy ready-to-consume meals, the increasing range of convenience foods for preparation at home reflects the changing social and cultural structures in many industrial countries. More people live alone, and more women work outside the home. On going technological developments make their contribution to our changing demands.

Meeting consumer demands in this new century is a big challenge in terms of safety, health, organoleptic, economic and sustainable aspects and will require further scientific and technological progress. Our awareness of the importance of a healthy diet and an active lifestyle parallels our growing scientific knowledge on the beneficial effects of various ingredients. The number of foods with scientifically proven health benefits will increase within the next decades, but they will not be a panacea for poor dietary habits. As the matter gets more and more complex, it will be very important to keep informed.

Functional foodstuffs

Functional foods may be conventional foods that are consumed in their natural state (like fruits, vegetables, grains) or novel foods that are modified or enriched with functional components to provide greater health benefits (like omega-3 eggs, phytosterol-enriched margarines). A functional foodstuff should be able to modify one or more organic functions favourably, in addition to its nutritional effect. For these products to be labelled as "nutraceutics" or "nutraceuticals", their therapeutic role should be demonstrated. These kinds of studies are of particular importance in the case of therapeutic claims against cancer and vascular diseases.

A precursor of nutraceutics is cod liver oil, which has greatly contributed to the control of rickets, a consequence of vitamin-D deficiency. In Europe and the USA, large-scale studies involving tens of thousands of volunteers are being carried out to determine the preventive action of vitamins A- and E-enriched substances and selenium-containing compounds on some pathological conditions resulting from the deficiency of these vitamins and selenium.

In the 1990s, the concept of the potential benefit of functional foodstuffs has become widespread, and the research carried out has led to its first products: an 'anticholesterol' oil, derived from maize; a rice deprived of its most allergenic properties; and a grapevine synthesising more resveratrol (an anti-oxidant well known for its impact on cardiovascular diseases).

Food science and biotechnology can lead to substantial innovations in the production of healthier foodstuffs as well as increased profits by major food companies. The modification of vegetable oils is one of the key areas of plant and crop biotechnology, the overall objective being to increase their content in unsaturated fatty acids (mainly oleic acid) and to decrease that of saturated ones through conventional breeding, induced mutations or genetic engineering. Extensive work has been carried out on oilseed rape (canola), soyabeans, peanut and sunflower with good results that led to the commercialisation of several products.

Palm oil, which contains an equal proportion of saturated and un-saturated fatty acids, in addition to betacarotene, is also a current research target, particularly of researchers at the Palm Oil Research Institute of Malaysia (PORIM). In addition, replacing triglycerides with diglycerides in vegetable oils render them free of trans-hydrogenated fats and good cooking oils, e.g. 'econa oil' in Japan. Inulin and oligofructosans refer to a group of fructosecontaining carbohydrate polymers (fructans) which, in many plant species, act as protective agents against dehydration and cold temperatures and also offer many health benefits to humans, mainly in the stimulation of the growth of beneficial micro-organisms called bifidobacteria.

These bacteria are sometimes used as a probiotic additive to foodstuffs such as yoghurt, as they can defeat harmful bacteria in the intestines and produce compounds with good health benefits. These dietary fructans are also reported to have a lipid-lowering potential. They are not digested in the upper gastro-intestinal tract and therefore have a reduced caloric value. They share the properties of dietary fibres without causing a rise in serum glucose or stimulating insulin secretion. Inulin and oligofructosans can be used to fortify foods with fibre or improve the texture of low-fat foods without resulting in adverse organoleptic effects. Most of these two products currently on the market are either chemically synthesised or extracted from plant sources such as chicory roots.

Oligofructosans are shorter chain polymers, highly soluble and provide 30 per cent to 50 per cent of the sweetness of sugar, and also have the other functional qualities of sugars. In formulation, inulin forms a smooth creamy texture, which makes this compound suitable as a fat substitute. Growers of nutraceutical plants need varieties with good agronomic potential and those that are consistent with the varieties in terms of germination time, height and maturity. Growers will need to be able to guarantee the quality of their natural health-beneficial products.

Breeding methods can therefore be used to achieve uniform quality for clinical testing and for product development, as well as to remove these potentially harmful or otherwise un-desirable compounds that are produced in the plants along with their therapeutic ones. To meet these goals, Alison Ferrie of the Plant Biotechnology Institute (PBI, National Research Council of Canada, Saskatoon, Saskatchewan) was using the doubled haploid technology or "haploidy", which facilitates the development of true-breeding lines.

Immature pollen grains, called microspores, were cultured to produce haploid lines, whose genetic stock was thereafter doubled. Truebreeding plants were thus produced in one generation, and doubled haploid techniques reduced the time required to develop a new variety by about three to four years. At the NRC-PBI, doubled haploid technology has been developed for oilseed rape (canola) and wheat. It is being applied to a wide range of nutraceutical and herbal species. Over 80 species have been screened for embryogenic response; anise, fennel, dill, caraway, angelica and lovage have shown good potential.

Haploidy could also be combined with mutagenesis to enhance the desirable components or decrease the undesirable characteristics. Mutagenising single cells (microspores) had definite advantages over seed mutagenesis. The new market for healthier foodstuffs attracts both the agri-food giants and pharmaceutical groups, so that the competition is harsh among them and the frontiers are less marked between both kinds of corporations. The competitive advantage of the food industry in this race is that it has a good knowledge of consumers' behaviour, massive marketing strategies while knowing that nutraceutics should remain tasteful and palatable if these were to be patronised by consumers.

In France, a success story was that of Danone's Actimel, launched in 1995 in Belgium in the form of a small bottle corresponding to an individual dose and commercialised in 15 countries. More than 600 million bottles had been sold worldwide in 1999, including about 100 million in France, where 9 per cent of the households of all socio-professional categories bought Actimel – dubbed the 'morning health gesture'. Others include that of the case of Eridania-Béghin Say in France in 1999, relating to food additives having an impact on cardiovascular diseases, colon cancer, osteoporosis, diabetes, etc. which sold commercialised powder sugar enriched with 'biofibres', which boosts intestinal microflora and helps the body to naturally resist illness.

Back in Nestlé, they are also carrying out the relevant research-and-development work with the support of its 600-scientists strong nutrition centres, located in

Lausanne while in May 1999, in the USA, Australia, and in Switzerland, Unilever with an international nutrition research centre at Vlaardingen, Netherlands, commercialised a 'hypocholesterol' margarine, which could help prevent the accumulation of 'bad' cholesterol. It also aimed to target markets in Europe and Brazil. In the USA, most agri-food companies (e.g. Campbell, Kellogg's and Quaker Oats) have developed soups, beverages and cereals, which can help digestion and prevent cardiovascular diseases and hypertension.

The US Food and Drug Administration (FDA) has opened the way to nutraceutics, having labels carrying a health recommendation. On 21 October 1999, the FDA granted to soyabeans (25 g. of soyabean proteins absorbed daily) the clearance to carry the claim 'may reduce cardiovascular risks' on their labels. This request was made by E.I. Dupont de Nemours & Co., Inc., the world's first-biggest producer of soyabean products. Soya sauce and soyabean paste are major foodstuffs across Asia. Industrial soyabeans undergo a solid-state fermentation process using compliant stainless steel tanks instead of in conventional bamboo trays.

They are also inoculated with Aspergillus oryzae selected strains that have been developed in Thailand to produce koji in higher yields and of better quality. This technique, developed by a fermentation consortium associating the National Center for Genetic Engineering and Biotechnology (BIOTEC, Bangkok) and the Department of Chemical Engineering of Kasetsart University (Agricultural University, Bangkok), has been successfully applied by the company Chain Co. Ltd., Bangkok, and thereafter adopted by some soya sauce manufacturers in Thailand. The same company has succeeded in selecting the appropriate strain of Lactobacillus to replace the addition of acetic acid in order to enhance the sour taste of soya sauce. The company produces the top quality commercial soya sauce in Thailand – the so-called First Formulation (the Thai Food and Drug Administration categorises soya sauce into five formulations which differ in protein content).

Long-chain polyunsaturated fatty acids

Long-chain polyunsaturated fatty acids are a research focus for nutritionists and food biotechnologists. Their beneficial effect on the functioning of the cardiovascular system has been initially mentioned since the 1970s in the medical literature. In France, a recent book authored by David Servan-Schreiber – a psychiatrist advocating a 'medicine of emotions' – Guérir le stress, l'anxiété et la dépression sans médicaments ni psychanalyse (Curing stress, anxiety and depression without medication or psychoanalysis) has stressed the role of these fatty acids as anti-depression substances. Incidentally, the author of the said book is also a share-holder of a company that sells pills containing these fatty acids.

These long-chain polyunsaturated fatty acids belong to two main categories: omega-3 (first double bound at carbon 3 on the chain) and omega-6 (first double bound at carbon 6 on the chain). Among omega-3 fatty acids, there are the alphalinolenic acid (ALA) with 18 carbon atoms, eicosapentaenoic acid (EPA) with 20 carbon atoms and docosahexaenoic acid (DHA) with 22 carbon atoms. The human body cannot synthesise the ALA as well as the linoleic acid which is an omega-6 fatty acid. Omega-3 fatty acids are found in rapeseed and soybean oils (linolenic acid), marine animals and human milk (EPA, DHA).

Food-consumption surveys carried out in France have shown that the consumption of omega-3 fatty acids was insufficient and the ratio of omega 6 to omega 3 was not balanced (this ratio should be between 5 and 10).

Although research is being carried out on the precise role of these fatty acids on human health, it is not easy for the public to have a clear view of established scientific facts and amid controversial statements. Let us look now at what may be causing confusion among the public as regard the issue of omega-3 fatty acids. It may have begun with the study that revealed lower morbidity and mortality due to cardiovascular of Greenland's Inuits who consume a lot of fattyfish.

Morbidity and mortality reduction was indeed significant among the persons who suffered form cardiovascular or metabolic diseases. However, omega-3 fatty acids did not act on cholesterol; they may act on triglycerides and cell membranes, as well as on blood clotting and heart excitability; they may also have, through prostaglandins (some of these acids are precursors in the biosynthetic pathways of prostaglandins), a positive effect on hypertension. The experts convened by the French AFSSA also warned against the role of the consumption of excessive quantities of omega-3 fatty acids, as they would increase cell susceptibility to free radicals.

They recommended a maximum daily intake of EPA and DHA of 2g per day. Then there are also the claims on the prohibitive effects of omega-3 fatty acids on tumors. To this, the AFFSA experts concluded that all the studies carried out up to 2004 on food habits did not sub-stantiate in humans any evidence indicating that an enrichment of the diet with precursors of omega-3 fatty acids would protect against cancer. However, research work carried out on rats has shown that a diet enriched with omega-3 fatty acids caused a 60 per cent decrease in size of mammary tumours, twelve days after radiotherapy, compared with a 31 per cent decrease in animals fed with a non-enriched diet.

Trials are expected to be carried out on humans. Given the insufficiency of evidence, the benefits of taking

Omega-3 pills remain inconclusive. In view of this, the general advice is to consume fish at least twice a week. The same goes for rapeseed oil. This is sufficient to meet the daily needs of omega-3 fatty acids. It is also recommended to feed poultry with rapeseed meal rather than with sunflower meal, because the former is richer in omega- 6 fatty acids. Thus, consuming this kind of poultry meat would provide enough omega-6 fatty acids.

Bio-fortification of Food Crops

Bio-fortification of food crops makes sense as part of an integrated food-systems approach to reducing malnutrition. It addresses the root causes of micronutrient deficiencies, targets the poorest people, and is scientifically feasible and cost-effective. It is a first step in enabling rural households to improve family nutrition and health in a sustainable way. Harvest Plus is a coalition of CGIAR Future Harvest Centers or Institutes, partners collaborating institutions and supportive donors.

The International Center for Tropical Agriculture (CIAT) and IFPRI are co-ordinating the plant breeding, human nutrition, crop dissemination, policy analysis and impact activities to be carried out at international Future Harvest Centers, national agricultural research and extension institutions, and departments of plant science and human nutrition at universities in both developing and developed countries. An initiative of the Consultative Group on International Agricultural Research (CGIAR), Harvest Plus is a global alliance of research institutions and implementing agencies coming together to breed and disseminate crops with improved nutritive value (bio-fortification), e.g. with a higher content of iron, zinc and vitamin A.

The bio-fortification approach is backed by sound science. Initial bio-fortification efforts will focus on six staple crops for which pre-breeding studies have been completed: beans, cassava, sweet potatoes, rice, maize and wheat. The potential for nutrient enhancement will also be studied in ten additional crops that are important components in the diets of those with micronutrient deficiencies: bananas/plantains, barley, cowpeas, groundnuts, lentils, millet, pigeon-peas, potatoes, sorghum and yams.

During the first four years (1 to 4) of the project, the objectives are to: determine nutritionally optimal breeding objectives; screen CGIAR germplasm for high iron, zinc and beta-carotene amounts; initiate crosses of high-yielding adapted germplasm for selected crops; document cultural and food-processing practices, and determine their impact on micronutrient content and bio-availability; identify the genetic markers available to facilitate the transfer of traits through conventional and novel breeding strategies; carry out in-vitro and animal studies to determine the bio-availability of the enhanced micronutrients in promising lines; and initiate bio-efficacy studies to determine the effect on biofortified crops on the micronutrient status of humans.

During the following three years (5 to 7), the objectives are to: continue bio-efficacy studies; initiate farmerparticipatory breeding; adapt high-yielding, conventionally-bred, micronutrient-dense lines to select regions; release new conventionally-bred bio-fortified varieties to farmers; identify gene systems with potential for increasing nutritional value beyond conventional breeding methods; produce transgenic lines at experimental level and screen for micronutrients, test for compliance with bio-safety regulations; develop and implement a marketing strategy to promote the improved varieties; and begin production and distribution.

During the last three years of the project (8 to 10), production and distribution of the improved varieties will be scaled up; the nutritional effectiveness of the programme will be determined; and the factors affecting the adoption of bio-fortified crops, the health effects on individuals and the impact on household resources will be identified. **The following are the staple crops and notes on their bio-tech status and potential:**

Rice

Rice is the dominant cereal crop in many developing countries and is the staple food for more than half of the world's population. In several Asian countries, rice provides 50 per cent to 80 per cent of the calorie intake of the poor. In South and South-East Asian countries, more than half of all women and children are anaemic; increasing rice nutritive value can therefore have significant positive health impact. Food-consumption studies suggested that doubling the iron content in rice could increase the iron intake of the poor by 50 per cent; germplasm screening indicated that a doubling of iron and zinc content in un-milled rice was feasible.

Milling losses vary widely by rice variety, with losses of iron being higher than losses of zinc, which suggests than more zinc is deposited in the inner parts of the rice endosperm. Under the Harvest Plus Project, improved rice germplasm will be provided to national partners in Bangladesh, Indonesia, Vietnam, India and the Philippines. The improved features will be incorporated into well-adapted and agronomically-preferred germplasm in ongoing breeding programmes at the national and regional level. A plant-bio-technology approach is the current priority for enhancing provitamin-A content of the rice endosperm. The leading varieties will be field tested for agronomic performance and compositional stability in at least four countries.

Wheat

The International Maize and Wheat Improvement Center (CIMMYT, Mexico) is leading the Harvest Plus research endeavour on wheat bio-fortification in order to increase people's intake of iron and zinc. Given that spring wheat varieties developed by CIMMYT and its partners are used in 80 per cent of the global spring wheat area, the potential impact of iron-enhanced wheat could be dramatic. The initial target countries will be Pakistan and India, in the area around the Indo-Gangetic plains, a region with high population densities and high micronutrient malnutrition.

The highest contents of iron and zinc in wheat grains are found in landraces of wild relatives of wheat such as Triticum dicoccon and Aegilops tauschii. Because these wild relatives of wheat cannot be crossed directly with modern wheat, researchers facilitated the cross between a high micronutrient wild relative, Aegilops tauschii, and a high micronutrient primitive wheat. Triticum dicoccon, to develop a variety of hexaploid wheat that can be crossed directly with current modern varieties of wheat and have 40 per cent to 50 per cent higher contents of iron and zinc in the grain than modern wheat. The first bio-fortified lines will be delivered to the target region by 2005, i.e. broadly-adapted, high-yielding, disease-resistant wheat lines.

The first high yielding lines with confirmed iron and zinc contents in the grain should be available for regional deployment by mid-2007. Researchers will be exploring the introduction of the ferritin gene in wheat and will establish the feasibility of increasing the concentration of iron and zinc in the grain using advanced bio-technology approaches in addition to conventional plant breeding. Molecular markers for the iron and zinc genes that control concentration in the grain were being identified in order to facilitate their transfer. Scientists will also carry out studies on bio-availability to determine the extent to which iron and zinc status in animal and human subjects is improved when bio-fortified varieties are consumed on a daily basis over several months.

Maize

Maize is the preferred staple food of more than 1.2 billion consumers in sub-Saharan Africa and Latin America. Over 50 million people in these regions were vitamin A-deficient in 2004. The International Maize and Wheat Improvement Center (CIMMYT) and the International Institute of Tropical Agriculture (IITA, Ibadan, Nigeria) are identifying micronutrient-rich maize varieties and will carry out adaptive breeding for local conditions in partnership with National Agricultural Research Systems (NARS) in Africa and Latin America. The project under HarvestPlus is initially focusing on maize varieties having increased contents of provitamin A because a useful range of genetic variation has already been identified for this trait.

The first target countries are Brazil, Guatemala, Ethiopia, Ghana and Zambia. To support the breeding programme, research is being conducted in Brazil, the USA and Europe to develop simple, inexpensive and rapid screening protocols for pro-vitamin A, so as to reduce the cost of assays from $70-100 to $5-10 per sample. Research in Brazil and the USA is also focused on finding genetic markers to facilitate marker-assisted selection for pro-vitamin A concentration. In collaboration with the University of Wageningen, a human efficacy trial was planned with pro-vitamin A-rich maize in Nigeria for 2005 in order to study pro-vitamin A retention or loss for different storage, processing and common cooking methods. To facilitate extension and dissemination of bio-fortified maize varieties, country teams will be formed in the target countries in order to conduct adaptive breeding research, farmer-participatory variety evaluations, nutritional advocacy and pro-motional activities.

Beans

Common beans (Phaseolus vulgaris) are the world's most important food legume, far more so than chickpeas, faba beans, lentils and cowpeas. For more than 300 million people, an inexpensive bowl of beans is the main meal of their daily diet. The focus of Harvest Plus research is on increasing the concentration of iron and zinc in agronomically superior varieties. Over 2,000 accessions from the International Center for Tropical Agriculture (CIAT, Cali, Colombia) gene-bank and several hundred collections of African landraces have been screened for their nutrient contents. While the average iron concentration in these varieties is about 55 mg. per kg., researchers have found varieties the content of which exceeds 100 mg per kg.

The eventual goals are to obtain favourable combinations for productivity and nutritional traits, double the iron concentration and increase zinc concentration by about 40 per cent. The first bred lines with 70 per cent higher iron will likely emerge in 2006, while lines with double concentration of iron are anticipated in 2008. The proportion of iron and zinc that can be absorbed from legumes such as common beans is typically low, due to anti-nutrients, specifically phytates and polyphenols, which normally bind to the iron and zinc, making them unavailable to the organism.

Research indicated that it might be possible to reduce polyphenol concentrations genetically, thereby improving iron bio-availability. In contrast, vitamin C is an iron-absorption enhancer because it binds to iron and prevents it from becoming attached to the iron-absorption inhibitors. Beans are often consumed with vegetables, including bean leaves with the potential of bean leaves as a source of vitamin C still to be explored.

Sweet Potato

Sweet potato is an important part of the diet in East and Central Africa where vitamin-A deficiency is wide-spread. About 40 varieties of sweet potato with high dry bio-mass and pro-vitamin-A content have been introduced to sub-Saharan Africa. Of these, 10 to 15 were being tested widely in different agro-ecological areas in some countries. Some original varieties, mainly local landraces, have been well accepted by farmers and were being distributed on a small scale.

The variation in pro-vitamin-A content of newly harvested roots can be as much as 45 per cent. Much of the pro-vitamin A appears to be retained during storage, food preparation and cooking. In the South African Resisto variety, the pro-vitamin-A activity of the boiled roots was between 70 per cent and 80 per cent of that of freshly harvested roots. Additional studies were to be carried out in 2004 to determine the pro-vitamin-A losses during food processing and cooking based on the usual practices found in East and Central Africa. A human bio-efficacy study using an organoleptically acceptable promising variety was planned for 2005, once the food processing studies were completed.

PRO-BIOTICS AND PRE-BIOTICS

Pro-biotics are microbial food ingredients that beneficially influence human health while pre-biotics are non-digestible carbohydrates such as fructo- and galacto-oligosaccharides. Pro-biotics have been used historically in different cultures in the form of fermented dairy foods, vegetables and cereals. Health effects of pro-biotics have been reported in the oral cavity, stomach, small and large intestine and the vagina. Although they consist mainly of lactic acid bacteria, bifidobacteria and yeasts have also been successfully used.

Pre-biotics are organic food components that exert healthpromoting effects by improving the characteristics of intestinalflora. Established effects of pre-biotics are dietary fibre-like effects such as anti-constipation, faecal bulking and pH reduction. The potential effects of pre-biotics are similar to those of pro-biotics, since a major mechanism for pre-biotics lies in the support of probiotics. The synergistic combination of both pro-biotics and pre-biotics is called symbiotics.

Pro-biotic lactobacilli are known to affect immunomodulation. The increased understanding of the molecular factors affecting immunomodulation and immunogenicity will allow the selection of pro-biotic strains, with enhanced protective or therapeutic effects. European researchers have targeted two types of intestinal diseases: inflammations such as inflammatory bowel disease and infections such as those caused by rotaviruses and Helicobacter pylori (associated with ulcers). Two specially-selected pro-biotics will be tested in long-term human clinical trials for their alleviating effects on inflammatory diseases, such as Crohn's disease and ulcerative colitis – immune-mediated diseases that result in chronic relapsing inflammation of the gut.

Delivering the health benefits of pro-biotics and pre-biotics to consumers depends essentially on their successful processing. Viability, stability and functionality of these ingredients must be maintained during processing, formulation and storage. The effects of processing pro-biotics are being explored by the European researchers and used to develop optimal process and formulation technologies. New processing techniques will be applied to the development of functionally enhanced pre-biotics and symbiotic combinations.

Nutri-geno-proteo-metabolo-mics Era

Before the biotech era, research on food and nutrition dealt with establishing the importance of carbohydrates, fats and proteins in our diet, and with identifying trace elements and vitamins that are essential for the enzymes mediating our metabolism, respectively. The biotech era we are now just entering, concerns the understanding of the effects on specific gene expression of certain compounds as we eat. A good example is that of the regulation of a diverse group of genes whose proteins, generally enzymes, tend to either directly or indirectly scavenge strong oxidants or to decrease the probability of production of strong oxidants; these proteins are referred to as phase-2 proteins and, since most of them are enzymes, they are commonly referred to as phase-2 enzymes.

Strong oxidants can damage DNA thereby resulting in mutations that may lead to cancer; they scavenge the endothelial-derived vascular relaxation factor nitric oxide thereby promoting hypertension; and they also activate kinase pathways that lead to inflammation. The phase-2 terminology comes from the terminology describing enzymes that metabolize xenobiotics:

Phase-1 enzymes being the mono-oxygenases, mostly cytochrome P450s, that convert the generally hydrophobic xenobiotics to strong electrophiles, while the phase-2 enzymes form water-soluble adducts by the addition of glutathiyl, glucuronosyl or sulphate groups. Since the phase-2 enzyme genes all have anti-oxidant response elements (AREs) in their promoter regions, any gene with an ARE in the promoter region is referred to as phase-2 protein (enzyme).

Phase-2 enzymes include the classical ones such as NAD(P)H: quinone oxireductase 1, glutathione S-transferases A, M and P families, UDP-glucuronosyl transferases, as well as the more recently defined phase-2 proteins: ferritin H and L chains; cystine/ glutamate antiporter, peroxiredoxin I, heme oxygenase 1; L-gamma-glutamyl-L-cysteine ligase, metallothioneins, etc. All these proteins directly or indirectly inhibit strong oxidant formation, e.g. ferritin through sequestering iron, or promote strong oxidant scavenging, e.g. NAD(P) H: quinone oxireductase. Phase-2 protein genes are coordinately upregulated through activation of an ARE in their promoter regions.

Phase-2 protein inducers can be found in our diet: kaempferol, a flavonoid present in high amounts in kale; a.avonoid fraction found in blueberries/cranberries; enterolactone, a metabolite of the principle lignan secoisolariciresinol diglucoside found in the flax seeds; ellagic acid found in strawberries and raspberries/ blackberries; the flavolignan silibinin obtained from milk thistle (Silybum marianum) fruit; sulforaphane, the isothiocyanate metabolite of the glucosinolate glucoraphanin. There is much evidence that dietary intake of such phase-2 protein inducers can increase phase-2 gene expression in a number of tissues and that such induction can decrease the incidence of chemically induced tumours.

At the Plant Biotechnology Institute (PBI, National Research Council of Canada, Saskatoon, Saskatchewan), Juurlink and colleagues are working on the phase-2 protein-inducing isothiocyanate derivatives of certain glucosinolates, 4-methylsulfinylbutyl glucosinolate, commonly known as glucoraphanin. The Canadian researchers have shown that dietary intake of glucosinolates that give rise to phase-2 protein inducing isothiocyanates can improve hypertension in the spontaneously hypertensive stroke-prone rats (SHRsp); in addition, oxidative stress and inflammatory changes in various tissues in the ageing SHRsp was down-regulated.

The NRC-PBI's researchers also examined the effects of administration of the flavonoid quercetin in a neurotrauma model. They found that quercetin administration after spinal cord injury promotes retention of function, correlated with decreased inflammation. Not only is quercetin a very selective kinase inhibitor, but it is also known to be a phase-2 protein inducer (although more than an order of magnitude higher concentration of quercetin is required for this activity than is the case for sulforaphane). In collaboration with Shawn Ritchie and Dayan Goodenowe, Juurlink has begun examination of the effect of broccoli sprouts containing glucosinolates that are converted into phase-2 protein gene-inducing isothiocyanates on the metabolic profile and they have seen pronounced effects in liver and other organs.

Modification of Food Tastes

A breakthrough in the food industry would be to offer healthier versions of popular foodstuffs without affecting the taste. If it succeeds to do so, grapefruit juice could be sweet without added sugar and potato chips flavourful with half the current content of salt. This kind of research could have applications in medicine manufacture. The compound, adenosine 5′-monophosphate or AMP, occurs naturally (in human breast milk, among other sources) and, when added to certain foodstuffs, including coffee and canned or bottled citrus juice, the company states, it blocks some of the acidic tastes from being felt by the tongue.

The finding of a bitter suppressor attracts all food companies, e.g. Coca-Cola Co., Kraft Foods and Solae, a soya-foods firm owned by E.I. Dupont de Nemours and Co., Inc., and Bunge have each expressed interest in flavour and taste bio-technology. Kraft Foods and Solae are Linguagen clients while Coca-Cola Co. has signed a research deal with Senomyx, another bio-technology company. Some research has focused on finding compounds that would trick the receptors on the tongue by accentuating or blocking certain elements in the food, allowing people to taste a cup of coffee without adding cream or sugar, or the sensation of full-fat in low-fat products.

Processed foods such as canned soups, sauces and snacks like potato chips contain high amounts of salt to mask the bitter tastes that result from the very hot cooking process. Soft drinks are sweetened to tone down the bitter taste of caffeine. Food and beverage companies are, on the other hand, very concerned, as a group, about health and nutrition because of all the reports on epidemic obesity, epidemic diabetes, cardiovascular diseases and hypertension. Hence the search for compounds that keep food tasty, minus salt, sugar and fat.

BEVERAGE AND FOOD QUALITY

Genetic Tagging

Species-specific DNA markers can be used to identify animal species such as commercial molluscs and crustaceans, which represent a high proportion of aquacultural species. For instance, in Thailand, at the National Center for Genetic Engineering and Biotechnology (BIOTEC) Marine Biotechnology Unit, species-specific markers based on 16S ribosomal DNA (rDNA) polymorphism have been developed for penaeid shrimps, tropical abalone and oysters. The black tiger shrimp (Penaeus monodon) is the most commercially important cultured species in Thailand. Because of outbreaks of diseases, the white shrimp (P. vannamei) has been introduced into Thailand and cultured commercially.

On the other hand, external characteristics of P. monodon and P. semisulcatus are similar, but the growth rate of the latter is approximately three times slower than that of the former. In addition, P. merguiensis larvae, which could not yet be successfully cultured, were sold as those of P.vannamei. Species-specific markers were therefore developed for identifying the aforementioned species and P. japonicus as well. These markers can be applied to ensure quality control by properly labeling traded shrimp larvae. Three species of tropical abalone are found in Thailand's waters: Haliotis asinina, H. ovina and H. varia.

However, H. asinina is the most productive one, as it provides the highest ratio (85 per cent) between meat weight and total weight. H. asinina specific markers based on 16S rDNA polymorphism have been developed in order to prevent supplying the wrong abalone larvae for the industry as well as to foster quality control of abalone products from Thailand. Oyster farming has shown rapid growth in Thailand over the last few years. Taxonomic difficulties relating to Thai oysters have had a limiting effect on the culture efficiency and development of their closed life cycle. Molecular genetic markers have therefore been developed to identify the three commercially cultured oysters, Crassostrea belcheri, C. iredalei and Saccostrea cucullata.

DNA Fingerprinting

Since 1990, US and French researchers have been trying to establish the phylogenetic tree of the varieties of grapevine grown throughout the world, using the fingerprinting technique. The research consists of analysing the structure of certain regions of the genome of some grapevine varieties and comparing it with that of other varieties, so as to establish possible phylogenetic relations. For this analysis, the DNA is extracted from young ground leaves, but also from fruits and branches. The results of this first research have been published in 1999 in the Science Journal. There are about 6,000 grapevine varieties cultivated worldwide.

In order to establish the origin of a variety, specialists used to rely on phenotypic traits, such as the morphology of leaves, berries and grapes. In this way, varieties could be grouped in a few families. DNA fingerprinting enables the researchers to go further. It appears that the current grapevine varieties are the remote offspring of the grapevines grown during the Antiquity around the Mediterranean, or during the European Middle Ages. The current varieties are the result of lengthy breeding activities, identification and comparison work, and stabilisation of the selected strains or lines.

Similarly, aged wines of the chenin variety resemble the Hungarian today. But more surprising than the discovery of that kinship among the four grapevine varieties, was the identity of one of the progenitors of the initial couple that gave rise to these varieties. Indeed, several historical elements were in favour of the creation of lines through the cross pollination between the pinot noir and the white gouais; these crosses have given birth – as proven by the fingerprinting analysis to the three white and red varieties grown for a long time in various French Provinces, and for some decades, in many regions of the globe.

The surprising aspect of this discovery was that the white gouais is almost unknown, although the vine specialists in Montpellier continue to grow it and to make wine form it for their own pleasure. However, this variety has played a key role in the origin of French viticulture, according to R. Dion in his Histoire de la vigne et duvin en France des origines au XIXe siècle (History of vine and wine in France from its origins to the 19th century). A document dated from the 12th century mentioned this variety as a lower-grade one; in 1338, the white gouais was found in Metz under the name of goez; at that time, instructions were given to eliminate this variety from all the Metz territory and to privilege only the white and black fromental, considered as higher-grade varieties.

The gouais was found in Paris during the 14th century and, owing to the expansion of the workers' population, it progressively replaced the pinot noir of Burgundy, which was a good variety of Parisian vineyards. The extension of the gouais was due to the wish of the winemakers to produce a cheaper wine. However, the phenomenon was limited to Paris and its suburbs; in the vineyards located away from the capital, the gouais was rejected, more noble grapevine varieties were used and contributed to the reputation of French viticulture.

For the US and French researchers, this variety which has played a key role in the history of vine and wine, is the same as the heunisch variety of Central Europe, introduced in Gaul by a Roman emperor originating from Dalmatia. In Montpellier, the French researchers participating in the joint study with the US scientists from the University of California, Davis, have tried to reproduce the breeding between the pinot noir and white gouais in order to seek confirmation of the genetic research. Other attempts were expected to widen even more the range of cultivated grapevine varieties, for both their fruits and wines derived from them. But this approach was hindered by a drastic regulation, which practically prohibits any venture of this kind, while non-French winemakers and vinegrowers could do it.

In Apulia, in the heel of the Italian boot, drawing on grapes grown by up to 1,600 small farmers in the area, a California wine consultant associated with another Italian wine consultant from Friuli (northeastern corner of the country) are producing and marketing wines that have scored a great success worldwide, with 2004 projected sales 15 times as big as those in 1998, the winery's first year. The wines are called A-Mano – handmade – and by far the best known is a robust red made from a once-obscure grape named primitivo.

Nowadays, primitivo can stand on its own feet. In addition to A-Mano primitivo, other high-quality primitivos are grouped in an organisation called the Academia dei- Racemi, not a true cooperative but an association in which each member makes his own wine and joins the others for marketing support and technical advice. Based in Manduria, between the old cities of Taranto and Lecce, the group includes value-for-money labels like Masseria Pepe, Pervini and Felline.

3

PATTERNS OF FOOD CONSUMPTION

Promoting healthy diets and lifestyles to reduce the global burden of non-communicable diseases requires a multisectoral approach involving the various relevant sectors in societies. The agriculture and food sector figures prominently in this enterprise and must be given due importance in any consideration of the promotion of healthy diets for individuals and population groups. Food strategies must not merely be directed at ensuring food security for all, but must also achieve the consumption of adequate quantities of safe and good quality foods that together make-up a healthy diet.

Economic development is normally accompanied by improvements in a country's food supply and the gradual elimination of dietary deficiencies, thus improving the overall nutritional status of the country's population. Furthermore, it also brings about qualitative changes in the production, processing, distribution and marketing of food. Increasing urbanisation will also have consequences for the dietary patterns and lifestyles of individuals, not all of which are positive. Changes in diets, patterns of work and leisure – often referred to as the "nutrition transition" – are already contributing to the causal factors underlying non-communicable diseases even in the poorest countries. Moreover, the pace of these changes seems to be accelerating, especially in the low-income and middle-income countries.

The dietary changes that characterise the "nutrition transition" include both quantitative and qualitative changes in the diet. The adverse dietary changes include shifts in the structure of the diet towards a higher energy density diet with a greater role for fat and added sugars in foods, greater saturated fat intake (mostly from animal sources), reduced intakes of complex carbohydrates and dietary fibre, and reduced fruit and vegetable intakes. These dietary changes are compounded by lifestyle changes that reflect reduced physical activity at work and during leisure time. At the same time, however, poor countries continue to face food shortages and nutrient inadequacies.

Diets evolve over time, being influenced by many factors and complex interactions. Income, prices, individual preferences and beliefs, cultural traditions, as well as geographical, environmental, social and economic factors all interact in a complex manner to shape dietary consumption patterns. Data on the national availability of the main food commodities provide a valuable insight into diets and their evolution over time. FAO produces annual Food Balance Sheets which provide national data on food availability (for almost all commodities and for nearly all countries).

Food Balance Sheets give a complete picture of supply (including production, imports, stock changes and exports) and utilisation (including final demand in the form of food use and industrial non-food use, intermediate demand such as animal feed and seed use, and waste) by commodity. From these data, the average per capita supply of macronutrients (i. e. energy, protein, fats) can be derived for all food commodities. Although such average per capita supplies are derived from national data, they may not correspond to actual per capita availability, which is determined by many other factors such as inequality in access to food.

Likewise, these data refer to "average food available for consumption", which, for a number of reasons (for example, waste at the household level), is not equal to average food intake or average food consumption. Actual food availability may vary by region, socio-economic level and season. Certain difficulties are encountered when estimating trade, production and stock changes on an annual scale. Hence three-years averages are calculated in order to reduce errors. The FAO statistical database (FAOSTAT), being based on national data, does not provide information on the distribution of food within countries, or within communities and households.

DIETARY ENERGY

Food consumption expressed in kilocalories (kcal) per capita per day is a key variable used for measuring and evaluating the evolution of the global and regional food situation. A more appropriate term for this variable would be "national average apparent food consumption" since the data come from national Food Balance Sheets rather than from food consumption surveys. Analysis of FAOSTAT data shows that dietary energy measured in kcals per capita per day has been steadily increasing on a worldwide basis; availability of calories per capita from the mid-1960s to the late 1990s increased globally by approximately 450 kcal per capita per day and by over 600 kcal per capita per day in developing countries (Table 1). This change has not, however, been equal across regions.

The per capita supply of calories has remained almost stagnant in sub-Saharan Africa and has recently fallen in the countries in economic transition. In contrast, the per capita supply of energy has risen dramatically in East

Asia (by almost 1000 kcal per capita per day, mainly in China) and in the Near East/North Africa region (by over 700 kcal per capita per day). In short, it would appear that the world has made significant progress in raising food consumption per person. The increase in the world average consumption would have been higher but for the declines in the transition economies that occurred in the 1990s.

Table 1: Global and regional per capita food consumption (kcal per capita per day)

Region	1964-1966	1974-1976	1984-1986	1997-1999	2015	2030
World	2358	2435	2655	2803	2940	3050
Developing countries	2054	2152	2450	2681	2850	2980
Near East and North Africa	2290	2591	2953	3006	3090	3170
Sub-Saharan Africa	2058	2079	2057	2195	2360	2540
Latin America and the Caribbean	2393	2546	2689	2824	2980	3140
East Asia	1957	2105	2559	2921	3060	3190
South Asia	2017	1986	2205	2403	2700	2900
Industrialized countries	2947	3065	3206	3380	3440	3500
Transition countries	3222	3385	3379	2906	3060	3180

It is generally agreed, however, that those declines are likely to revert in the near future. The growth in food consumption has been accompanied by significant structural changes and a shift in diet away from staples such as roots and tubers towards more livestock products and vegetable oils. Table 1 shows that current energy intakes range from 2681 kcal per capita per day in developing countries, to 2906 kcal per capita per day in transition countries and 3380 kcal per capita per day in industrialised countries.

Globally, the share of dietary energy supplied by cereals appears to have remained relatively stable over time, representing about 50% of dietary energy supply. Recently, however, subtle changes appear to be taking place (Fig. 1).

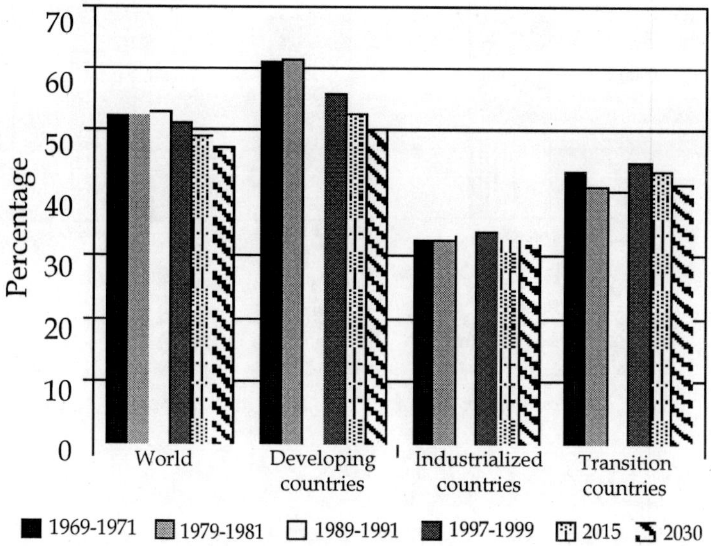

Figure 1: The Share of Dietary Energy Derived from Cereals

A closer analysis of the dietary energy intake shows a decrease in developing countries, where the share of energy derived from cereals has fallen from 60% to 54% in a period of only 10 years. Much of this downwards trend is attributable to cereals, particularly wheat and rice, becoming less preferred foods in middle-income countries such as Brazil and China, a pattern likely to continue over the next 30 years or so. Fig. 2 shows the structural changes in the diet of developing countries over the past 30–40 years and FAO's projections to the year 2030.

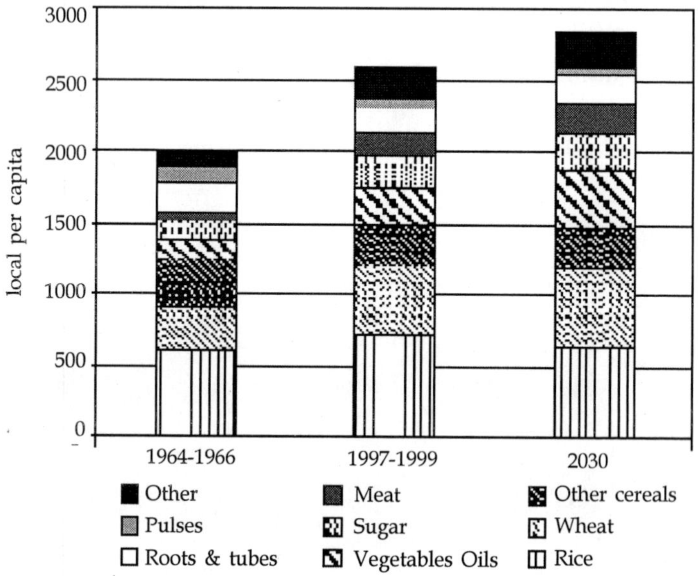

Figure 2: Calories from Major Commodities in Developing Countries

DIETARY FAT

The increase in the quantity and quality of the fats consumed in the diet is an important feature of nutrition transition reflected in the national diets of countries. There are large variations across the regions of the world in the amount of total fats (i.e., fats in foods, plus added fats and oils) available for human consumption. The lowest quantities consumed are recorded in Africa, while the highest consumption occurs in parts of North America and Europe. The important point is that there has been a remarkable increase in the intake of dietary fats over the past three decades and that this increase has taken place practically everywhere except in Africa, where consumption levels have stagnated.

The per capita supply of fat from animal foods has increased, respectively, by 14 and 4 g per capita in developing and industrialised countries, while there has been a decrease of 9 g per capita in transition countries. The increase in dietary fat supply worldwide exceeds the increase in dietary protein supply. The average global supply of fat has increased by 20 g per capita per day since 1967–1969. This increase in availability has been most pronounced in the Americas, East Asia, and the European Community. The proportion of energy contributed by dietary fats exceeds 30% in the industrialised regions, and in nearly all other regions this share is increasing.

The fat-to-energy ratio (FER) is defined as the percentage of energy derived from fat in the total supply of energy (in kcal). Country-specific analysis of FAO data for 1988–1990 found a range for the FER of 7–46%. A total of 19 countries fell below the minimum recommendation of 15% dietary energy supply from fat, the majority of these being in sub-Saharan Africa and the remainder in South Asia. In contrast, 24 countries were above the maximum recommendation of 35%, the majority of these countries being in North America and Western Europe.

It is useful to note that limitations of the Food Balance Sheet data may contribute much of this variation in the FER between countries. For instance, in countries such as Malaysia with abundant availability of vegetable oils at low prices, Food Balance Sheet data may not reflect real consumption at the individual household level. Rising incomes in the developing world have also led to an increase in the availability and consumption of energy-dense high-fat diets. Food balance data can be used to examine the shift in the proportion of energy from fat over time and its relationship to increasing incomes.

In 1961—1963, a diet providing 20% of energy from fat was associated only with countries having at least a per capita gross national product of Rs. 66375. By 1990, however, even poor countries having a gross national product of only Rs. 33750 per capita had access to a similar diet comprising 20% of energy from fat. This change was mainly the result of an increase in the consumption of vegetable fats by poor countries, with smaller increases occurred in middle-income and high-income countries. By 1990, vegetable fats accounted for a greater proportion of dietary energy than animal fats for countries in the lowest per capita income category.

Changes in edible vegetable oil supply, in prices and in consumption equally affected rich and poor countries, although the net impact was relatively much greater in low-income countries. An equally large and important shift in the proportion of energy from added sugars in the diets of low-income countries was also a feature of the nutrition transition. Examinations of the purchasing habits of people, aimed at understanding the relationship between level of education or income and the different amounts or types of commodities purchased at different times were also revealing.

Research conducted in China shows that there have been profound shifts in purchasing practices in relation to income over the past decade. These analyses show how extra income in China affects poor people and rich people in a differential manner, enhancing the fat intake of the poor more than that of the rich. A variable proportion of these fat calories are provided by saturated fatty acids. Only in the two of the most affluent regions (i. e. in parts of North America and Europe) is the intake of saturated fat at or above 10% of energy intake level.

In other less affluent regions, the proportion of dietary energy contributed by saturated fatty acids is lower, ranging from 5% to 8%, and generally not changing much over time.

National dietary surveys conducted in some countries confirm these data. The ratio of dietary fat from animal sources to total fat is a key indicator, since foods from animal sources are high in saturated fat. Data sets used to calculate country-specific FERs can also be used to calculate proportions of animal fat in total fat. Such analysis indicated that the proportion of animal fat in total fat was lower than 10% in some countries (Democratic Republic of Congo, Mozambique, Nigeria, Sao Tome and Principe, and Sierra Leone), while it is above 75% in some other countries (Denmark, Finland, Hungary, Mongolia, Poland and Uruguay). These findings are not strictly divided along economic lines, as not all of the countries in the high range represent the most affluent countries. Country-specific food availability and cultural dietary preferences and norms to some extent determine these patterns.

The types of edible oils used in developing countries are also changing with the increasing use of hardened margarines (rich in trans fatty acids) that do not need to be refrigerated. Palm oil is becoming an increasingly important edible oil in the diets of much of South-East Asia and is likely to be a major source in the coming years. Currently, palm oil consumption is low and the FER ranges between 15% and 18%. At this low level of consumption, the saturated fatty acid content of the diet comprises only 4% to 8%. Potential developments in the edible oil sector could affect all stages of the oil production process from plant breeding to processing methods, including the blending of oils aimed at producing edible oils that have a healthy fatty acid composition.

Olive oil is an important edible oil consumed largely in the Mediterranean region. Its production has been driven by rising demand, which has increasingly shifted olive cultivation from traditional farms to more intensive forms of cultivation. There is some concern that the intensive cultivation of olives may have adverse environmental impacts, such as soil erosion and desertification. However, agricultural production methods are being developed to ensure less harmful impacts on the environment.

ANIMAL PRODUCTS

There has been an increasing pressure on the livestock sector to meet the growing demand for high-value animal protein. The world's livestock sector is growing at an unprecedented rate and the driving force behind this enormous surge is a combination of population growth, rising incomes and urbanisation. Annual meat production is projected to increase from 218 million tonnes in 1997–1999 to 376 million tonnes by 2030. There is a strong positive relationship between the level of income and the consumption of animal protein, with the consumption of meat, milk and eggs increasing at the expense of staple foods. Because of the recent steep decline in prices, developing countries are embarking on higher meat consumption at much lower levels of gross domestic product than the industrialised countries did some 20–30 years ago.

Urbanisation is a major driving force influencing global demand for livestock products. Urbanisation stimulates improvements in infrastructure, including cold chains, which permit trade in perishable goods. Compared with the less diversified diets of the rural communities, city dwellers have a varied diet rich in animal proteins and fats, and characterised by higher consumption of meat, poultry, milk and other dairy products. Table 2 shows

Table 2: Per capita consumption of livestock products

Region	Meat (kg per year)			Milk (kg per year)		
	1964-1966	1997-1999	2030	1964-1966	1997-1999	2030
World	24.2	36.4	45.3	73.9	78.1	89.5
Developing countries	10.2	25.5	36.7	28.0	44.6	65.8
Near East and North Africa	11.9	21.2	35.0	68.6	72.3	89.9
Sub-Saharan Africa	9.9	9.4	13.4	28.5	29.1	33.8
Latin America and the Caribbean	31.7	53.8	76.6	80.1	110.2	139.8
East Asia	8.7	37.7	58.5	3.6	10.0	17.8
South Asia	3.9	5.3	11.7	37.0	67.5	106.9
Industrialized countries	61.5	88.2	100.1	185.5	212.2	221.0
Transition countries	42.5	46.2	60.7	156.6	159.1	178.7

trends in per capita consumption of livestock products in different regions and country groups.

There has been a remarkable increase in the consumption of animal products in countries such as Brazil and China, although the levels are still well below the levels of consumption in North American and most other industrialised countries. As diets become richer and more diverse, the high-value protein that the livestock sector offers improves the nutrition of the vast majority of the world. Livestock products not only provide high-value protein but are also important sources of a wide range of essential micronutrients, in particular minerals such as iron and zinc, and vitamins such as vitamin A.

For the large majority of people in the world, particularly in developing countries, livestock products remain a desired food for nutritional value and taste. Excessive consumption of animal products in some countries and social classes can, however, lead to excessive intakes of fat. The growing demand for livestock products is likely to have an undesirable impact on the environment. For example, there will be more large-scale, industrial production, often located close to urban centres, which brings with it a range of environmental and public health risks. Attempts have been made to estimate the environmental impact of industrial livestock production.

For instance, it has been estimated that the number of people fed in a year per hectare ranges from 22 for potatoes and 19 for rice to 1 and 2, respectively, for beef and lamb. The low energy conversion ratio from feed to meat is another concern, since some of the cereal grain food produced is diverted to livestock production. Likewise, land and water requirements for meat production are likely to become a major concern, as the increasing demand for animal products results in more intensive livestock production systems.

CONSUMPTION OF FISH

Despite fluctuations in supply and demand caused by the changing state of fisheries resources, the economic climate and environmental conditions, fisheries, including aquaculture, have traditionally been, and remain an important source of food, employment and revenue in many countries and communities. After the remarkable increase in both marine and inland capture of fish during the 1950s and 1960s, world fisheries production has levelled off since the 1970s. This levelling off of the total catch follows the general trend of most of the world's fishing areas, which have apparently reached their maximum potential for fisheries production, with the majority of stocks being fully exploited. It is therefore very unlikely that substantial increases in total catch will be obtained in the future.

In contrast, aquaculture production has followed the opposite path. Starting from an insignificant total production, inland and marine aquaculture production has been growing at a remarkable rate, offsetting part of the reduction in the ocean catch of fish. The total food fish supply and hence consumption has been growing at a rate of 3.6% per year since 1961, while the world's population has been expanding at 1.8% per year. The proteins derived from fish, crustaceans and molluscs account for between 13.8% and 16.5% of the animal protein intake of the human population.

The average apparent per capita consumption increased from about 9 kg per year in the early 1960s to 16 kg in 1997. The per capita availability of fish and fishery products has therefore nearly doubled in 40 years, outpacing population growth. As well as income-related variations, the role of fish in nutrition shows marked continental, regional and national differences. In industrialised countries, where diets generally contain a more diversified range of animal proteins, a rise in per capita provision from 19.7 kg to 27.7 kg seems to have occurred. This represents a growth rate close to 1% per year. In this group of countries, fish contributed an increasing share of total protein intake until 1989 (accounting for between 6.5% and 8.5%), but since then its importance has gradually declined and, in 1997, its percentage contribution was back to the level prevailing in the mid-1980s.

In the early 1960s, per capita fish supply in low-income food-deficit countries was, on average, only 30% of that of the richest countries. This gap has been gradually reduced, such that in 1997, average fish consumption in these countries was 70% of that of the more affluent economies. Despite the relatively low consumption by weight in low-income food-deficit countries, the contribution of fish to total animal protein intake is considerable (nearly 20%). Over the past four decades, however, the share of fish proteins in animal proteins has declined slightly, because of faster growth in the consumption of other animal products. Currently, two-thirds of the total food fish supply is obtained from capture fisheries in marine and inland waters, while the remaining onethird is derived from aquaculture.

The contribution of inland and marine capture fisheries to per capita food supply has stabilised, around 10 kg per capita in the period 1984–1998. Any recent increases in per capita availability have, therefore, been obtained from aquaculture production, from both traditional rural aquaculture and intensive commercial aquaculture of high-value species. Fish contributes up to 180 kcal per capita per day, but reaches such high levels only in a few countries where there is a lack of alternative protein foods grown locally or where there is a strong preference for fish (examples are Iceland, Japan and some small island states).

More typically, fish provides about 20–30 kcal per capita per day. Fish proteins are essential in the diet of some densely populated countries where the total protein intake level is low, and are very important in the diets of many other countries. Worldwide, about a billion people rely on fish as their main source of animal proteins. Dependence on fish is usually higher in coastal than in inland areas. About 20% of the world's population derives at least one-fifth of its animal protein intake from fish, and some small island states depend almost exclusively on fish.

Recommending the increased consumption of fish is another area where the feasibility of dietary recommendations needs to be balanced against concerns for sustainability of marine stocks and the potential depletion of this important marine source of high quality nutritious food. Added to this is the concern that a significant proportion of the world fish catch is transformed into fish meal and used as animal feed in industrial livestock production and thus is not available for human consumption.

FRUITS AND VEGETABLES

Consumption of fruits and vegetables plays a vital role in providing a diversified and nutritious diet. A low consumption of fruits and vegetables in many regions of the developing world is, however, a persistent phenomenon, confirmed by the findings of food consumption surveys. Nationally representative surveys in India, for example, indicate a steady level of consumption of only 120-140 g per capita per day, with about another 100 g per capita coming from roots and tubers, and some 40 g per capita from pulses. This may not be true for urban populations in India, who have rising incomes and greater access to a diverse and varied diet. In contrast, in China, – a country that is undergoing rapid economic growth and transition — the amount of fruits and vegetables consumed has increased to 369 g per capita per day by 1992.

At present, only a small and negligible minority of the world's population consumes the generally recommended high average intake of fruits and vegetables. In 1998, only 6 of the 14 WHO regions had an availability of fruits and vegetables equal to or greater than the earlier recommended intake of 400 g per capita per day. The relatively favourable situation in 1998 appears to have evolved from a markedly less favourable position in previous years, as evidenced by the great increase in vegetable availability recorded between 1990 and 1998 for most of the regions. In contrast, the availability of fruit generally decreased between 1990 and 1998 in most regions of the world. The increase in urbanisation globally is another challenge.

Increasing urbanisation will distance more people from primary food production, and in turn have a negative impact on both the availability of a varied and nutritious diet with enough fruits and vegetables, and the access of the urban poor to such a diet. Nevertheless, it may facilitate the achievement of other goals, as those who can afford it can have better access to a diverse and varied diet. Investment in periurban horticulture may provide an opportunity to increase the availability and consumption of a healthy diet. Global trends in the production and supply of vegetables indicate that the current production and consumption vary widely among regions. It should be noted that the production of wild and indigenous vegetables is not taken into account in production statistics and might therefore be underestimated in consumption statistics.

In 2000, the global annual average per capita vegetable supply was 102 kg, with the highest level in Asia (116 kg), and the lowest levels in South America (48 kg) and Africa (52 kg). These figures also include the large amount of horticultural produce that is consumed on the farm.

AVAILABILITY OF FOOD IN FUTURE

In recent years the growth rates of world agricultural production and crop yields have slowed. This has raised fears that the world may not be able to grow enough food and other commodities to ensure that future populations are adequately fed. However, the slowdown has occurred not because of shortages of land or water but rather because demand for agricultural products has also slowed. This is mainly because world population growth rates have been declining since the late 1960s, and fairly high levels of food consumption per person are now being reached in many countries, beyond which further rises will be limited.

It also true that a high share of the world's population remains in poverty and hence lacks the necessary income to translate its needs into effective demand. As a result, of growth in world demand for agricultural products is expected to fall from an average 2.2% per year over the past 30 years to an average 1.5% per year for the next 30- years. In developing countries the slow down will be more dramatic, from 3.7% per year to 2% per year, partly as a result of China having passed the phase of rapid growth in its demand for food. Global food shortages are unlikely, but serious problems already exist at national and local levels, and may worsen unless focused efforts are made. The annual growth rate of world demand for cereals has declined from 2.5% per year in the 1970s and 1.9% per year in the 1980s to only 1% per year in the 1990s.

Annual cereal use per person (including animal feeds) peaked in the mid-1980s at 334 kg and has since fallen to

317 kg. The decline is not a cause for alarm, it is largely the natural result of slower population growth and shifts in human diets and animal feeds. During the 1990s, however, the decline was accentuated by a number of temporary factors, including serious economic recessions in the transition countries and in some East and South-East Asian countries. The growth rate in the demand for cereals is expected to rise again to 1.4% per year up until 2015, slowing to 1.2% per year thereafter. In developing countries overall, cereal production is not expected to keep pace with demand.

The net cereal deficits of these countries, which amounted to 103 million tonnes or 9% of consumption in 1997–1999, could rise to 265 million tonnes by 2030, when they will be 14% of consumption. This gap can be bridged by increased surpluses from traditional grain exporters, and by new exports from the transition countries, which are expected to shift from being net importers to being net exporters. Oil crops have seen the fastest increase in area of any crop sector, expanding by 75 million hectares between the mid-1970s and the end of the 1990s, while cereal area fell by 28 million hectares over the same period.

Future per capita consumption of oil crops is expected to rise more rapidly than that of cereals. These crops will account for 45 out of every 100 extra kilocalories added to average diets in developing countries between now and 2030. There are three main sources of growth in crop production: expanding the land area, increasing the frequency at which it is cropped (often through irrigation), and boosting yields. It has been suggested that growth in crop production may be approaching the ceiling of what is possible in respect of all three sources.

Diets in developing countries are changing as incomes rise. The share of staples, such as cereals, roots and tubers, is declining, while that of meat, dairy products and oil crops is rising. Between 1964–1966 and 1997–1999, per capita meat consumption in developing countries rose by 150% and that of milk and dairy products by 60%. By 2030, per capita consumption of livestock products could rise by a further 44%. Poultry consumption is predicted to grow the fastest. Productivity improvements are likely to be a major source of growth.

Milk yields should improve, while breeding and improved management should increase average carcass weights and off-take rates. This will allow increased production with lower growth in animal numbers, and a corresponding slowdown in the growth of environmental damage from grazing and animal wastes. In developing countries, demand is predicted to grow faster than production, resulting in a growing trade deficit. In meat products this deficit will rise steeply, from 1.2 million tonnes per year in 1997–1999 to 5.9 million tonnes per year in 2030 (despite growing meat exports from Latin America), while in the case of milk and dairy products, the rise will be less steep but still considerable, from 20 million tonnes per year in 1997–1999 to 39 million tonnes per year in 2030.

An increasing share of livestock production will probably come from industrial enterprises. In recent years, production from this sector has grown twice as fast as that from more traditional mixed farming systems and more than six times faster than that from grazing systems. World fisheries production has kept ahead of population growth over the past three decades. Total fish production has almost doubled, from 65 million tonnes in 1970 to 125 million tonnes in 1999, when the world average intake of fish, crustaceans and molluscs reached 16.3 kg per person. By 2030, annual fish consumption is likely to rise to some 150–160 million tonnes, or between 19–20 kg per person. This amount is significantly lower than the potential demand, as environmental factors are expected to limit supply.

During the 1990s the marine catch levelled out at 80–85 million tonnes per year, and by the turn of the century, three-quarters of ocean fish stocks were overfished, depleted or exploited up to their maximum sustainable yield. Further growth in the marine catch can only be modest. Aquaculture compensated for this marine slowdown, doubling its share of world fish production during the 1990s. It is expected to continue to grow rapidly, at rates of 5–7% per year up to 2015. In all sectors of fishing it will be essential to pursue forms of management conducive to sustainable exploitation, especially for resources under common ownership or no ownership.

4

FUNCTIONAL FOODS AND NATURAL HEALTH PRODUCTS

In the past, foods were recognised as being nutritious based on their content of essential nutrients (fat, protein, carbohydrate, minerals and vitamins) that are needed for normal metabolic activity and bodily function. In recent years however, a growing body of scientific evidence has demonstrated that other food constituents (often referred to as phytochemicals and zoochemicals, when they come from plant and animal foods, respectively) may provide health benefits beyond basic nutrition and help prevent chronic diseases like cardiovascular disease, cancer and osteoporosis among others.

Examples of such disease-fighting food constituents include omega-3 fatty acids from fish, flaxseed, soyabean, hempseed and canola oil, isoflavones from soya beans, carotenoids (like beta-carotene and lycopene) from carrots, tomatoes and other red/orange fruits and vegetables, sulforophane from broccoli, polyphenols from tea and wine and soluble fibre from oats and barley. Foods that may have physiological benefits and/or have the ability to reduce the risk of chronic disease beyond basic nutritional functions are called functional foods. Functional foods may be conventional foods that are consumed in their natural state (like fruits, vegetables, grains) novel foods that are modified or enriched with functional components to provide greater health benefits (like omega-3 eggs, phytosterol-enriched margarines). Other words that are often used to describe functional foods include health foods, medical foods, designer foods, foods for special dietary use and pharmafoods.

Some functional foods have been scientifically proven to provide health benefits beyond basic nutrition. For many others however, the supporting evidence is only preliminary in nature. Unfortunately, it can take several years and millions of dollars for the purported health benefits of a functional food to be substantiated by scientific evidence. Although some functional foods may provide health benefits, no single food is a "magic bullet" for maintaining health and preventing disease. Consuming a balanced diet consisting of a variety of foods is the best way to maintain optimal health.

SAFETY OF FUNCTIONAL FOODS

Generally speaking, functional foods are considered safe to use. Many functional foods are conventional foods that have been consumed for hundreds of years without any significant safety concerns. Novel foods that have been modified in some way to convey a functional benefit must undergo a thorough safety assessment before they can be sold. Despite the apparent safety of functional foods however, some may have the potential to be hazardous, particularly when consumed in excess. Before making any major dietary changes, it is important to consult with a health care provider, especially if you are nursing or pregnant, have a chronic disease, are taking prescription medications or are about to undergo surgery. Once again, it must be emphasised that no single food is a "magic bullet" for maintaining health and preventing disease. A balanced diet consisting of a variety of foods is the safest and healthiest way to maintain optimal health.

NUTRACEUTICALS

Nutraceuticals are products that are isolated or purified from foods and generally sold in medicinal forms not usually associated with food (tablets, capsules, drops) that may have physiological benefits and/or have the ability to reduce the risk of chronic disease beyond basic nutritional functions. Examples of nutraceuticals include fish oils, soya isoflavones and canola phytosterols. Since nutraceuticals are sold in medicinal form and not consumed as food, they are often classified as natural health products.

Natural health products are naturally occurring substances that are consumed for the purpose of diagnosing, treating or preventing illness or maintaining or promoting health. Natural health product substances include plant, algal, fungal, or animal materials or extracts thereof; vitamins; minerals; amino acids; essential fatty acids and probiotics. They are usually sold in dosage form (capsule, pills, tablets or liquid extracts). The natural health product definition includes traditional medicines and homoeopathic preparations but excludes drugs and foods, among other substances. Since nutraceuticals are sold in medicinal form, they are sometimes classified as natural health products.

In the United States, the term 'dietary supplements' is used in place of natural health products. There is generally a need for further research to substantiate the purported health benefits of natural health products. For some natural health products, the scientific evidence is strong, but still inconclusive. For many others, the evidence is only preliminary in nature. Moreover, the chemical compositions and biological mechanisms of many natural health products are still poorly understood. Many natural health products vary significantly in chemical composition and therefore cannot be expected to produce consistent therapeutic effects.

B-COMPLEX VITAMINS

B-complex vitamin products provide several or all of the B-vitamins, but unlike multivitamins they do not contain other nutrients. Often, the B-vitamins are included at relatively high potencies, and the product may have names like "B-complex 100" or "B-complex 50," hinting at their composition of 100 mg or 50 mg of each of several of the B-vitamins. Selection of a B-complex mixture rather than a multivitamin or multivitamin with minerals presupposes a need for or benefit from the B-vitamins but not from other nutrients. There is little to no evidence that such a supposition is correct.

A rationale frequently offered for use of a B-complex mixture is that these vitamins are necessary for energy metabolism. While it is generally true that several of B-vitamins are involved in energy production, some are not. Vitamin B-6 is also involved in metabolism of amino acids and many other substances. Folic acid and vitamin B-12 are involved in production of DNA and RNA, among other actions.

Effects on Health: Marginal or deficient intakes of each of the B-vitamins are not equally likely to occur. The RDAs of vitamins B-1, B-2, and B-6 are similar. The RDA for niacin is much more, nearly 20 mg/day, and that for B-12 is much less, only 2 mcg/day. There is no rationale for taking all of the B-vitamins in equal amounts. Obtain B-vitamins from a wide variety of foods and a multivitamin with minerals.

BETA-CAROTENE

Beta-carotene is one of a group of compounds called

carotenoids that are part of the red, yellow, and orange pigments found in plant foods. Beta-carotene is a precursor of vitamin A. It is well known for its antioxidant properties. Beta-carotene is found in dark green leafy vegetables and yellow-orange fruits and vegetables.

Epidemiological studies during the past 25 years have indicated that diets high in carotenoid-rich fruits and vegetables, as well as high serum levels of beta-carotene, are associated with a reduced risk for several chronic diseases including heart disease, cataracts, and some cancers. However, three large-scale clinical trials concluded that beta-carotene provided no protection against lung cancer or cardiovascular disease. There is also evidence that the antioxidant activity of beta-carotene and other carotenoids at very high levels may shift into pro-oxidant activity inducing oxidative stress.

Dietary Recommendation: There is no dietary reference intake for beta-carotene and other carotenoids because the research is not sufficient to support any recommendation at this time. Strenuous exercise increases oxygen consumption with an increase in the production of free radicals. Beta-carotene may protect tissues against oxidative damage. In most studies involving exercise induced lipid peroxidation, beta-carotene was used in combination with other antioxidants such as vitamin E and vitamin C, making it difficult to determine if beta-carotene or other substances are responsible for any positive effects.

Supplement Range:

a) Athletes who habitually consume low levels of antioxidants may be at greater risk for the harmful effects of free radicals.

b) Athletes should be encouraged to eat a balanced diet that includes frequent servings of carotenoid-rich fruits and vegetables.

c) While mega doses or long term supplementation of beta-carotene is not warranted, there is no evidence that small amounts of supplemental beta-carotene is harmful to any population, including athletes.

MULTIVITAMINS WITH MINERALS

Multivitamin products have several advantages as sources of supplemental nutrients, they provide a wide spectrum of nutrients in generally appropriate proportions and ratios, and they give reasonable confidence that the total intake of a specific nutrient is not inadequate because of improper variations in food intake. The term "multivitamins" is not specific, but many such products are formulated to contain a very wide spectrum of vitamins and essential minerals. Products that contain both multiple vitamins and multiple minerals provide the greatest assurance that the total intake of each vitamin or mineral meets established nutritional need for that nutrient.

Similarly, the words "high potency" and numerous similar terms do not have specific meanings. Federal regulations allow use of "high potency" on the label if two-thirds of the nutrients included are at 100 percent or more of the Daily Value (DV). Some products are labeled "high potency" for this reason, even though a few of the nutrients are present only 10 to 25 percent of the DV because of their bulk (such as calcium) or cost (such as biotin). Many products labeled "high potency," "mega," "ultra," "maximum strength" or the like contains some of the vitamins at 100 to 300 percent or so of the DV. Many multivitamin/mineral products contain substances that may be nutritionally useful or even essential, but for which no DV has been established. These are listed only with an amount per day, rather than a percent DV.

Although the typical diet provides adequate amounts of many nutrients and perhaps surplus amounts of some, marginal intakes of certain nutrients are common among some sport groups. Nutrient intakes less than the DV usually do not indicate clinical deficiency, but the intakes are marginal and improvement of the diet or supplementation are needed to remove any risk of deficiency. Further more, intakes at the recommended level of several nutrients may not be adequate for persons at risk of deficiency-those with increased needs or nutrient losses. Anyone considering taking vitamin and mineral supplements must decide on multivitamins/minerals, individual nutrient supplements, or both. For convenience and lower cost, multivitamin/mineral products offer a broad array of nutrients at modest doses, and without taking a large number of tablets or capsules.

For high intakes of specific vitamins or minerals, multi- products generally are not a good approach. Nutrients such as calcium or vitamin E may be present in relatively low amounts that make it difficult to achieve the relatively high intakes that many persons want. Multivitamin/mineral products are an excellent way to assure maintenance intakes of vitamin A, vitamin D, most of the B-vitamins, and most minerals. The multivitamin should be checked to make sure that it contains at least 0.4 mg (400 mcg) of folic acid. The Food and Nutrition Board recommends 400 mcg of folic acid from fortified foods and/or supplements to reduce the risk of neural tube defects in women of child-bearing age.

Helpful intakes of some vitamins and minerals can be best obtained through supplements that contain only that nutrient, or perhaps a mixture of a few. Vitamin E intakes of 100 to 800 IU are impossible to get from conventional foods and are in very few multivitamins. Vitamin C intakes of 100 to 1,000 mg can be obtained from conventional foods if the diet is selected for that purpose (lots of citrus fruits, etc.), but some people find doing this every day can be difficult. Calcium intakes of 1,000 to 1,300 mg can be obtained from consistently high intakes of milk and milk products (about 5 servings per day), but many people cannot routinely achieve this.

Some nutrients are formulated into simple "multi" mixtures such as calcium with vitamin D, calcium with a few other minerals, or antioxidant products that might contain vitamin E, selenium, vitamin D, and some carotenes or a few other substances. These simple formulas and single-nutrient supplements can be conveniently used to achieve high intakes of targeted nutrients.

Dietary Recommendation

a) Consume a diet based on a wide variety of foods in accordance with the Food Guide Pyramid.

b) Consume a multivitamin/multimineral supplement providing 100 percent of the DV.

NIACIN

Niacin is required for energy metabolism (burning of fats, carbohydrates, amino acids, and alcohol), and for the synthesis and processing of many essential substances by the human body. The term "niacin" may be used specifically to describe nicotinic acid, but may also include "niacinamide" (nicotinamide). Niacin activity can be provided by its synthesis from the amino acid tryptophan. Sixty milligrams of tryptophan provides 1 mg of nicotinic acid, and thus typical dietary protein intakes provide 5 to 7 mg of "niacin equivalents." The RDA is 14 mg per day for women and 16 mg per day for men. Niacin is an appropriate component of multivitamins and B-complex supplements.

Nicotinic acid (but not nicotinamide) is an effective drug for lowering blood lipids and cholesterol when given at doses of several thousand milligrams. Nicotinic acid (but not nicotinamide) doses of approximately 50 mg or higher may cause a flushing reaction (vasodilation) that can be uncomfortable but is not hazardous. Gradual increases in intake may prevent this reaction.

Intakes that are effective as a cholesterol-lowering drug carry a recognisable risk of substantial side effects (gastrointestinal distress and liver effects). Therapeutic doses should be avoided unless under proper medical supervision and monitoring. Slow-release forms of nicotinic acid have greater potency as a drug and potential for adverse effects. Persons taking crystalline (not slow-release) niacin in doses of 50 mg or more should be aware of the flushing reaction.

The two coenzyme forms of niacin, NAD and NADP, participate in numerous metabolic activities and are central in energy production from carbohydrates, amino acids and fatty acids, as well as glycogen synthesis. A deficiency has the potential to affect both muscular and nervous function. Studies have shown that supplementation with niacin in high doses can suppress free fatty acid release through decreased lipolysis. This in turn, can result in a decreased availability of a major fuel source, causing the muscles to reply more on its glycogen stores which may impair prolonged exercise performance.

There is no evidence that the requirement for niacin is increased in exercise, and there is no need for niacin supplementation in exercise.

a) Consume foods rich in niacin (e.g., enriched cereals, pasta, meats, chicken and peanut butter).

b) Take a multivitamin that includes 100 percent of the DV for niacin.

c) Be aware of the potential side effects with higher doses.

Selenium: Selenium may help prevent cancer and possibly heart disease. In early 2002, USDA's Agricultural Research Service launched a study to research moderately high doses of selenium and their effects on human cardiovascular health, immune function, and reproductive health. More than 30 healthy men aged 18-45 are participating in the study. For one year, half the volunteers will take a daily capsule providing five and one-half times the recommended dietary allowance of selenium in the form of high-selenium yeast. The other half will receive a daily placebo-a capsule containing only yeast and no selenium.

Samples of blood, urine, semen, and other specimens will be provided for laboratory tests at regular intervals. Participants will also receive tests for cardiovascular function and several other health indicators. In addition, they will complete detailed records of their exercise, general health, and the foods they have eaten during specific 3-day periods. It is hoped that the project, already in its second phase, will provide new, detailed information about selenium. device level, linked to Profibus at the intermediate level and to Ethernet at the highest level.

Almost all modern instruments come with some network protocol built in, whether it is used or not. Most smart process instruments are HART-compatible. A food plant may need to integrate several protocols to accommodate the convey or heavy and discrete device-heavy packaging area with the more process-oriented areas of a plant. In this respect, a food plant can require a more challenging control system than much larger process plants in which the nature of information is more uniform. The food industry has been relatively slow to adopt some of these technologies, according to those experts charged with introducing these technologies to food companies. In part, this is because there have not been many new food plants built, but it may also be because the industry is only now beginning to appreciate the advantages offered by the various networks. As older plants are replaced or upgraded, the control systems will become smarter and more sophisticated.

Safety of Natural Health Products

Natural health products whose chemical compositions and biological mechanisms are well understood can be standardised to contain specific amounts of active constituents, and can therefore be expected to produce consistent therapeutic effects. Despite a lack of scientific evidence to substantiate their purported benefits and inconsistency in chemical composition and quality, natural health products can still be sold under current laws and regulations, provided that they are safe and that they do not bear any unsubstantiated drug-like claims (claims of treating or preventing illness or disease) on their labels.

Instead of drug claims, manufacturers are often use indirect and often misleading "general well-being" statements that are not always substantiated by scientific evidence. Many natural health products have been used as traditional remedies for hundreds of years and are therefore presumed to be safe. Moreover, natural health products usually produce much fewer adverse side effects than conventional drugs. Despite their historical use and low incidence of adverse effects however, it should not be assumed that all natural health products are safe. There is often a lack of scientific data proving the safety of natural health products in the context in which most North Americans are using them today.

There have been a number of instances when natural health products have been removed from the market due to severe adverse events, some of which were attributed to interactions with conventional drugs. There have also seen instances when natural health products have been contaminated with pharmaceuticals and other foreign agents. In Canada, products bearing drug identification numbers (DIN) on their labels are manufactured in accordance with strict drug standards and are therefore less likely to be contaminated than products that do not bear DINs. Due to the potential hazards of using natural health products it is important to consult with a health care provider before beginning self-treatment, especially if you are nursing or pregnant, have a chronic disease, are taking prescription medications or are about to undergo surgery.

A growing body of scientific evidence suggests that functional foods and natural health products have the potential to contribute significantly to health maintenance and disease treatment and prevention. Although the safety and efficacy of some of these products have been substantiated with scientific evidence, for many others, the evidence is only preliminary in nature. Furthermore, there are a number of problems and inconsistencies with the developing North American functional foods/ natural health product industry that must be resolved before the true benefits of functional foods and natural health products can be realised. As laws and regulations improve and research continues to separate fact from fiction, functional foods and natural health products are likely to play an increasingly important role in health maintenance and disease prevention in coming years.

PROPERTIES OF FIGS

Functional foods is still evolving but refers to "foods that, by virtue of physiologically active components, provide benefits beyond basic nutrition and may prevent disease or promote health. Increasingly, manufacturers are including the names of non-nutritive components on their labels. The public is becoming more knowledgeable about these non-nutritive ingredients because of the large amount of publicity and articles in the mass media.

Today there is an ever increasing demand for foods that will increase our intake of food components that are perceived to be "protective against disease." In the future, genetic engineering will allow us to provide a variety of fruit or vegetables that is highly elevated in a certain compound. One example of such research is the work by the USDA and others in the development of a tomato high in lycopene, a carotenoid understood to be an antioxidant and anticancer substance.

In some varieties, the concentration of lycopene can be three times that of regular tomatoes. The genes responsible for the synthesis of carotenoids such as lycopene have been isolated. The genes have been inserted in an edible yeast and have produced lycopene and carotenoid at 0.1% dry weight of isolated cells. We are increasingly using foods as preventive agents to decrease our risk of deadly chronic diseases, including cancer and heart disease.

Figs (Ficus Carica) are one of the earliest fruits cultivated. Figs were dried and stored for later consumption. There was a fig tree in the Garden of Eden, and the fig is the most mentioned fruit in the Bible. Figs are mentioned in a Babylonian hymnbook dated about 2000 B.C. As early as 2900 B.C., in early Sumerian times, the medical use of figs was already being stressed. Legend has it that the Greek goddess Demeter first revealed to mortals the fruit of autumn, which they called the fig. It was the favourite fruit of Cleopatra, and she ended her life with an asp brought to her in a basket of figs.

Every inhabitant of Athens was a "philosykos,"

literally translated, "a friend of the fig." Early Olympic athletes were given figs as a training food and figs were given as laurels to the winners of the first Olympics as a "medal". The Wildlife Conservation Society of New York has recently determined that, in the animal and plant kingdom, the high-calcium content of wild figs makes them a "keystone" fruit, critical to the survival of other plants and animals.

Although considered a fruit, the fig is actually a flower inverted into itself. The seeds are the real fruit in figs. They are the only fruit to ripen fully and semidry on the tree. Native to areas from Asiatic Turkey to northern India, figs spread to all the countries around the Mediterranean. Today the United States, Turkey, Greece, and Spain are the primary producers of dried figs. The Spaniards brought figs to the Americas in the early 16th century. The missionary fathers brought them to California where they were planted from San Diego to Sonoma.

"Mission Fig" gets its name from this history. The Smyrna fig was imported from Turkey to California in 1882. It was given the hybrid name of Calimyrna in honour of the grower's home. California, specifically the San Joaquin Valley, produces 100% of the dried figs grown in the United States. Fig trees reach fruit-bearing age in one to two years and have tremendous longevity.

Some trees planted at the beginning of California's commercial fig production are still bearing fruit almost 100 years later. There are four principal varieties of cultivated figs: the amber-coloured Calimyrna; the dark, purplish Mission; the small but high-in-sugar Adriatic, and the uniquely white-totranslucent amber Kadota. The Calimyrna and Mission varieties represent almost two-thirds of the commercial production.

Dried figs are available in many forms: whole for the consumer and, in industrial products, as paste, concentrate, nuggets, powder, and diced forms. Potassium sorbate is added to dried figs to inhibit yeast fermentation and mold growth. Dried figs are processed to bring their moisture content up from 14-20% to as high as 30%. Compared to other dried fruits such as apricots or apples, colour in the Calimryna variety may be stabilised by the addition of low levels of sulfur dioxide.

NUTRIENT COMPOSITION OF DRIED FIGS

One serving of figs is 100gl., about ¼ cup, or about three Calimyrna or four to five Mission figs. Figs are fat free, sodium free and, like other plant foods, cholesterol free. Of the common fruits, figs have the highest overall content of minerals, and their calcium content per serving is second to oranges. Figs provide more fiber than all of the common fruits. A single serving contains 20% of the daily value of fiber. More than 28% of the fiber is the soluble variety. Soluble fiber has been shown to help control blood sugar and lower blood cholesterol by binding to it in the digestive tract.

The addition of a soluble-fiber supplement to the diet can aid in weight loss. Pasman studied obese women and found that average energy intake decreased significantly after fiber supplementation while hunger and satiety scores did not change. In a second study of subjects with low-energy intakes, hunger scores were significantly decreased after fiber supplementation. The authors concluded that, by facilitating compliance to a low-energy intake, fiber may be useful in the treatment of obesity.

Thus, figs and their soluble fiber may be of help with weight reduction, particularly considering the recent finding that over half of Americans, 97 million people, are overweight and 23% are grossly overweight, i.e., obese.

The upward trend in adult obesity seen in the last 40 years has also been observed in children. Figs, as both a fruit and a snack, are an ideal addition to a child's diet and an adult's because they represent an excellent source of fiber and are naturally sweet.

Reducing the Risk of Cancer

It has been estimated that up to 70% of the incidences of cancers are related to diet. Major dietary hypotheses relate high fat consumption to breast and colorectal cancers; high alcohol intake to respiratory, gastrointestinal, breast, and liver cancers; and low fiber intake to colorectal cancer. Of course 128 of 156 epidemiological studies have shown an inverse correlation between the consumption of fruits and vegetables and the incidence of cancer.

There was a substantial reduction in risk for all cancers among those consuming a large amount of fruits and vegetables. Previously, it was thought that the antioxidant vitamins, vitamin C, E, and b carotene, were responsible for the beneficial effects of fruits and vegetables as shown by epidemiology studies across many cultures.

However, recent supplement studies have been disappointing with respect to that hypothesis. For instance, a Cancer Institute study on male smokers was halted because it was found that 5-8 years of vitamin E supplementation had no benefit. b carotene supplementation, in fact, was correlated with a significant increase in the incidence of lung cancer. No effect of supplementation with the antioxidants vitamin C, E, or Coenzyme Q10 was found with respect to oxidative DNA damage in smokers.

Out of almost 200 epidemiological studies, the relationship between cancer risk and fruit and vegetable intake is exceptionally strong and consistent. People who eat greater amounts of fruits and vegetables have about one-half the risk of getting cancer and have less mortality from cancer. It is the hypothesis of many scientists that the polyphenols in the fruits and vegetables are responsible for the reduced cancer-risk benefits they offer.

The polyphenols can act by several mechanisms to prevent cancer, such as carcinogen- blocking activities, antioxidant and free-radical scavenging, and antiproliferation/ antiprogression actions. In test tube studies, five classes of polyphenols were tested for their ability to inhibit the binding of the potent carcinogen benzopyrene to DNA in liver cells. These compounds were active after being fed to rats and subsequent exposure of the rats' liver cells to the carcinogen.

At least 22 studies have been conducted in which cancer has been experimentally induced (usually by means of a chemical carcinogen or irradiation) in animals fed vegetables or fruits. In most of these studies, it has been unequivocally found that the animals experienced fewer tumors, smaller tumors, fewer metastases, less DNA damage, higher levels of enzymes involved in the detoxification of carcinogens, or other outcomes indicative of lower cancer risk.

For an example, in one study, rats were given a diet with and without a vegetable-fruit mixture. The rats were exposed to a high-fat diet and a chemical carcinogen that induced colorectal cancer. Rats fed high-fat diets developed significantly more tumors than did rats fed low-fat diets, which indicates the underlying importance of a low-fat diet for lowering the risk of cancer. Also, a lower number of tumors were found in the rats fed vegetables and fruits along with the fat and a carcinogen.

Besides their ubiquitous polyphenols, figs have

other compounds with anticancer activity, specifically benzaldehyde and the coumarins. Benzaldehyde has been used successfully to treat terminal human carcinomas. Of 57 evaluable patients, 19 responded completely and 10 responded with a greater than 50% regression in their cancers when treated with benzaldehyde. Treatment of squamous cell carcinomas with benzaldehyde induced the cancer cells to change into keratinized, normal squamous cells.

Coumarins are the major compounds isolated from the volatile extract of figs. In fact, the total dry-weight coumarinic content of figs is 0.5%. The furanocomarins identified in figs include angelicin, marmesin, psoralen, umbelliferone, and bergapten. Coumarins have also been used for the treatment of prostate cancer. Among cancers, the incidence of skin cancer is currently growing at the fastest rate.

The age standardised rates for melanoma have increased 60% compared to the rates in the 1970s, with the greatest proportional increase occurring among younger age groups. Psoralens, such as the fig compound angelicin, are currently being investigated for the treatment of skin cancer and have been recommended for clinical trials because they have low skin phototoxicity. These compounds produce free radicals and photoadducts of DNA that inhibit proliferation of the cancer cells.

Heart Diseases

Elevated lipids such as cholesterol and triglycerides are risk factors for developing heart disease, the number one cause of death in the United States. The public knows that a low-fat diet high in fiber is beneficial with respect to reducing the risk of heart disease. However, another causal mechanism related to metabolism and the transport of lipids needs to be explained.

Lipids are water-insoluble nutrients, but they are transported through the body by the blood. This is achieved by the lipids' "packaging" in water-soluble particles of lipoprotein. In these lipoproteins, the amphiphatic lipids (phospholipids and some non-esterified cholesterol) and the receptor protein are on the outside of the particles. The hydrophobic lipids (cholesteryl esters, triglycerides and some non-esterified cholesterol) are protected from water in the interior of the particles.

The four main types of lipoproteins are chylomicrons, very low-density lipoprotein (VLDL), low-density (LDL) and highdensity lipoproteins (HDL). Chylomicrons transport triglycerides mainly from the small intestine to the adipose tissue and skeletal muscle, while VLDL transports triglycerides mainly from the liver to the adipose tissue and skeletal muscle. In the circulation, VLDL is converted to LDL.

Each LDL particle is about 22 mm in diameter on average and contains in its core about 1,800 oxidizable molecules in the form of cholesteryl esters and triglycerides. There are about 700 molecules of phospholipid on the LDL particle's surface as a monolayer and approximately 600 molecules of non-esterified cholesterol distributed between its core and its surface. LDL's antioxidant defence is contained within the particle and consists of about 20 molecules, mostly the phenolic vitamin E tocopherol with minor amounts of carotenoids and coenzyme Q10.

The oxidative theory of atherogenesis was first promulgated in Steinberg's seminal paper in 1989. The hypothesis states that it is not LDL or VLDL that is atherogenic but the oxidized form of these lipoproteins.

LDL and VLDL enter the arterial wall from the plasma and are oxidized locally within the wall by oxidizing agents derived from cells, such as macrophages, smooth muscle cells, endothelial cells, and lymphocytes. The oxidized LDL and VLDL are then believed to bind to scavenger receptors on macrophages and internalised rapidly by receptor-mediated endocytosis.

The amount of cholesterol from the lipoproteins entering the cells overwhelms the capacity of the macrophages to release it, and the cholesterol accumulates inside the cells and converts them to foam cells, which are the first visible evidence of atherosclerosis. This hypothesis has been substantiated by many different pieces of evidence both in vitro and in vivo.

There is overwhelming epidemiological evidence of the protective effect of vegetables and fruits against heart disease and, as has been recently found, stroke. A highly significant negative association between the consumption of total fresh fruits and vegetables and ischemic heart disease was reported in the United Kingdom and in the United States. A significant negative relationship between fruit and vegetable consumption and stroke in men was recently found in the Dutch Study. An additional benefit of fruits and vegetables are their negative association with blood pressure, a risk factor for heart disease.

The first indication that flavonoids could function as protection against heart disease came in a study published in the famous 1979 Lancet article, which, using data from 17 countries, showed an inverse relationship between coronary artery-disease mortality and wine drinking. This led researchers to examine the so-called "French paradox," which describes the apparent contradiction in the data on the French, where a very low incidence of heart disease and mortality, as compared with North Americans, exists alongside the same average serum cholesterol, saturated fat intake, blood pressure, and prevalence of smoking found in countries with high rates of heart disease.

It was hypothesised that the French's much greater intake of wine was responsible for this effect. Because, in France and the other countries studied, red wine is normally consumed at meals, it was natural to assume that the flavonoids were responsible for this effect, since red wines have a high polyphenol content. Similarly, wine ethanol had the strongest and most consistent negative correlation with coronary heart disease mortality in 21 developed countries.

The first epidemiological report indicating that the intake of antioxidant flavonols (as measured in the diet by an HPLC method) reduced the rate of coronary heart disease mortality was released in 1993. The five-years study on elderly Dutch men also reported that intakes of tea, onions, and apples were inversely related to coronary heart disease mortality. A strong inverse association between flavonol plus flavone intake and mortality from coronary heart disease. The composite diets of 1987 were analysed and used for the correlation study.

In multivariate analysis flavonoids explained 8% of the variance in heart disease rates. In fact, saturated fat and smoking plus flavonoids explained 90% of the variance in heart disease rates, independent of alcohol and antioxidant vitamin intake. A Finnish study with a 26-years followup period showed a significant inverse gradient between dietary intake of flavonoids and total and coronary mortality. Between the lowest and highest quartile of dietary flavonoids intake, there was a 31% lower risk of total mortality and a 48% lower risk of coronary mortality.

For men, there was a 34 and 32% lower risk, respectively. Apple and onion consumption were inversely associated with total and coronary mortality. A recently completed epidemiological study of male health professionals in the United States found a modest but non-significant inverse association between intake of flavonols and flavones and subsequent coronary mortality rates. The risk was 37% lower for those the highest quintile of intake of flavonoids compared with those in the lowest.

Elderly male population, a study of 552 men followed up for 15 years, dietary flavonoids were inversely associated with incidence of stroke, after adjustment for potential confounders in the data, including antioxidant vitamins. Black tea consumption was inversely associated with incidence of stroke. The intake of vitamin C and vitamin E was not associated with stroke risk.

Polyphenols in Nuts, Cereals, Fruits, Vegetables, and Beverages One limitation to these types of studies is that the methodology for determining polyphenol intake generally underestimates the polyphenol content; therefore, this error is carried over to the analyses in these epidemiological studies. Using an acidhydrolysis and HPLC separation, Hertog measured the total aglycone content of five flavonols and flavones in nine fruits and 28 vegetables and beverages. Using this assay method, it was found that the average U.S. diet contains 20 mg/day of these five compounds.

Thus, only five compounds out of the 4,000 known natural substances were used in the epidemiological methodology. Kühnau estimated the intake of polyphenols to be about 1 g/day.The quantity of total polyphenols was measured in dried figs after an acid hydrolysis to liberate the free phenols and polyphenols and followed by reaction with the Folin-Cocialteu reagent, which assays oxidizable polyphenols versus a catechin standard.

Using 100 g as a comparison, it is evident on a weight basis that figs contain one of the highest concentrations of polyphenols among the commonly consumed foods and beverages. Only barley, some sorghums, and some beans have the same high levels found in figs. Compared with figs, red wine and tea, two well known and well-publicised sources of polyphenols, are low in phenols. Putting it in perspective, 40 g of figs, the suggested serving size, provide an average of 444 mg of phenols, which is more than the daily per capita consumption of polyphenols from vegetables or 218 mg/day.

5

HEALTH, NUTRITION AND DAIRY PRODUCTS

Food is functional if it contains a food component that affects one or a limited number of functions in the body. Functional food could be naturally occurring food, not just enriched or modified food. The diet-health message has reached consumers and the food industry. Consumers are beginning to believe that diet has a powerful influence on health and wellbeing and the food industry has taken advantage of new possibilities.

Progress in food processing and biotechnology has enabled the food industry to create food with special characteristics and in addition to disease prevention, the role of food as an agent for improving health has been proposed. New terms such as probiotics, prebiotics, synbiotics and functional food have been created to describe food products with special characteristics.

Many chronic diseases such as cancer, osteoporosis, coronary heart disease and hypertension are connected to an unbalanced diet. There are many aspects of functional food and as a consequence term has no exact definition. It is usually described as "food which promote health beyond providing basic nutrition". Milk itself is much more than the sum of its nutrients. The development of an infant's immature physiological functions is very dependent on milk and therefore is logical that milk is a natural source of a variety of beneficial nutrients and biologically-active compounds with a potential impact on human health.

Pro-biotic bacteria beneficially affect the host improving the properties of in-testinal microbial balance. Pro-biotic effects include alleviation of intestinal disorders such as lactose intolerance, acute gastroenteritis due to rotavirus and other enteric pathogens, adverse effects of pelvic radiotherapy, constipation, inflammatory bowel disease, and food allergy.

Besides functional food, on the market we also find a group of foods described as "lesser evil foods", which include foods with the negative properties removed (foods free of or with reduced levels of fat, cholesterol, salt or sugar). Many products that might be considered functional already exist in nature, although their health benefits have not ever been emphasised.

DIET-HEALTH MESSAGE

Consumers have got the message about the relationship between diet and health and believe that the three most important factors contributing to health are diet, exercise and genetic factors. In European research programme performed in 1993 it was found that diet was perceived to be the most important factor, cited by 70 % of respondents in Germany, 68 % of UK respondents and 55 % of French respondents, well ahead of exercise and genetic factors.

An increasing number of people believe that specific foodstuffs contain active substances which reduce the danger of illness and which generally contribute to the improvement of one's health. These foods are attractive to modern men and women who desire to reach old age in a healthy and vital state. An excessively simplistic interpretation of scientific findings regarding the link between diet and health can lead to entirely mistaken judgements or conclusions, based either on fear or on hope.

It is interesting that in popular magazines the number of articles which discuss the harmful effects of foodstuffs or (even more often) their ingredients, and which therefore scare the reader, is much higher than the number of articles dealing with the healthy and beneficial effects of food, and which are aimed at raising public awareness. This most likely results from the fact that the area of education is the responsibility of experts, who usually find it difficult to present generally complex scientific findings in a simple and concise manner.

This particularly applies to multi- disciplinary fields of interest such as food. On the other hand, articles which discuss the harmful effects of "toxicity" and the danger of consuming specific foodstuffs are frequently written by unqualified persons; this is reflected in the factual errors (the result of misconceptions, rather than misprints) which often pervade articles written by these authors and which point to their lack of knowledge.

It is also interesting that alarming statements such as those on the harmfulness of milk fat and proteins tend to stick in people's minds more than positive statements, as, for example, explanations of probiotic bacteria. Most people are familiar with the harmful effects of fats and cholesterol, and with the link between them and coronary heart disease. As a result, even if it is not necessary, they resort to consuming low-fat products and preparations which reduce cholesterol.

There are only a few people who know what probiotics are, not to mention functional food. The great majority of consumers opt for this food mainly because they read "bio" or "natural" on the label, and assume it is therefore likely to be healthier. The genuine experts, are partly to blame for this because we often tend to look only through our own eyes, forgetting that our discoveries are merely a small piece of the mosaic which will ultimately – and only when all the pieces are put together – explain the significance of a specific foodstuff in our diet.

Consumers are familiar only with the harmful effects of milk fat, while it is much less known that scientists are currently discovering the important roles played by a number of ingredients in milk fat, such as conjugated linoleic acid, butyric acid, anti-oxidants, and vitamins soluble in fat. Additionally, it is possible that determinants of healthful effects of dairy product are multifactorial, for example due to live bacteria and other components of fermented milk such as highly absorbable calcium, conjugated linoleic acid and bioactive peptides.

Isolation of a single component may not yield the positive benefits of a whole food. Important nutritional qualities of milk are the wide range of nutrients it contains and the good balance of its nutrients. Therefore to define the value of dairy foods in a healthy diet above all in the light of complex interactions between milk components and their combined effect on organism. Three common chronic diseases will be taken by way of example.

MILK, DAIRY PRODUCTS AND CARDIOVASCULAR DISEASE

Coronary heart disease (CHD), the most common and serious form of cardiovascular disease, is the leading cause of death in developed industrialised countries. Many risk factors, both genetic and environmental, contribute to the development of this disease. It is evident that diet is an important modifiable risk factor. Obesity, dietary fat quantity, particularly those with increased fat content. However, there is little evidence from scientific studies that dairy foods contribute to an atherogenic blood profile when consumed in usual amounts. Interpretation of such results was that "the biological basis for this observation is unknown and it may be due to factors in the lifestyle of people who choose to drink milk regularly, rather than to a protective factor in milk as such".

There are protective factors in milk and possible mechanisms which could explain such observations. Milk fat has often been characterised as containing a high proportion of saturated fatty acids but it needs to be added that only three of them, representing about one third of the milk fatty acids, are cholesterolemic. These are lauric (12:0), myristic (14:0) and palmitic (16:0) acid. Furthermore, milk and dairy products contain components with at least a protective if not hypoholesterolemic effect such as calcium, linoleic acid, conjugated linoleic acid (CLA), anti-oxidants and lactic acid bacteria or probiotic bacteria.

Calcium plays an important role in mediating vascular contraction and vasodilatation, muscle contraction, nerve transmission and glandular secretion. There are more and more proof that linoleic acid is beneficial in reducing CHD risk in human subjects, and some evidence that CLA protects against the development of early arterial lipid accumulation and helps regulate body weight and fat distribution.

It is well established that a raised level of serum cholesterol does not adequately explain the increased risk of CHD or the relationship between diet and CHD. Several lines of evidence indicate that the development of atherosclerosis is related to free radical processes, lipid peroxidation and oxidative modifications of low density lipoproteins (LDL).

LDL is the principal carrier of cholesterol but its atherogenic potential arises from an increase in the number of LDL particles and not from its cholesterol content per se. The oxidation of LDL promotes the final deposition of cholesterol in the arterial wall. It has been shown that LDL particles are more susceptible to oxidative modification than larger and lighter ones.

Fortunately, the cell possesses highly efficient protective mechanisms, including anti-oxidants such as -tocopherol, ascorbat, -carotene, glutathione, and metal-binding proteins such as transferrin and enzymes such as superoxide dismutase and catalase. The majority of this substances could be found also in milk and milk products.

Although pro-biotics, in the form of fermented milk products, have the reputation of cholesterol-lowering properties in humans, no conclusive evidence is available, with many studies giving conflicting results. The conflicting reports may be explained by factors such as differences in experimental design, species and strains of bacteria used as well as lifestyle and genetic or biochemical variability within and between human population.

Advances in genetics and molecular biology indicate that susceptibility to chronic diseases such as coronary artery disease, hypertension, diabetes, osteoporosis and cancer is to a great extent genetically determined.

Hypertension

Hypertension is another modern day problem and again both genetic and environmental factors influence blood pressure. People with high blood pressure are at increased risk of coronary heart disease, stroke, and kidney failure. Because of the high cost of the medicines and potential adverse side effects associated with pharmacological therapy for these diseases, people are encouraged to change their lifestyle from "harmful to healthy". This means weight reduction if overweight, increased physical activity, limited alcohol and sodium intake and adequate consumption of calcium, potassium, and magnesium.

Current scientific evidence indicates that it is not only an excess of one electrolyte (sodium) in our diets but rather inadequate levels of several, that produce hypertension. An adequate intake of calcium, potassium, and magnesium have now been documented to reduce blood pressure. Therefore, there is nothing surprising in the results found in several clinical trials that the effect of milk on blood pressure was greater and more rapid than that of calcium alone.

Milk and dairy products are meaningful sources of all three nutrients along with bioactive peptides termed casokinins or ACE – I peptides with a potential to reduce blood pressure due to their ability to inhibit angiotensin-I-converting enzyme (ACE) and block conversion of angiotensin I to angiotensin II, a potent vasoconstrictor.

Colon Cancer

Colorectal cancer is one of the leading causes of cancer morbidity and mortality in the Western countries and it is thought to be caused by an interaction between dietary factors and genetic predisposition. Diet is estimated to be responsible for 30 to 60 percent of all cancers but the role of diet in cancer etiology is difficult to elucidate because food contains components that may either cause or prevent cancer.

Epidemiological studies indicate that increased consumption of fat, meat, and total calories and low intake of foliate, fiber, and calcium enhance the risk of colon cancer but there are also several scientific proofs supporting the protective role of milk products. The components in dairy foods which may protect against colon cancer are above all calcium and vitamin D, probiotic lactic acid bacteria, a class of fatty acids known as conjugated derivatives of linoleic acid (LCA) and bioactive peptides derived from milk proteins.

A potential mechanism for the protective effect of calcium against colon cancer was suggested from animal studies. Dietary fat increases levels of bile acids and free fatty acids in the colonic lumen which damage the colonic epithelium and promote epithelial proliferation. Calcium binds and precipitates unconjugated bile acids and free fatty acids and thus its cytotoxicity is diminished.

The results of a randomized, double-blind, placebo-controlled clinical study which did not support this thesis. 193 subjects with a history of sporadic adenomatous polyps were treated with placebo (n = 66) or 1.0 g calcium (n = 64) or 2.0 g calcium (n = 63) daily for 6 months. Rectal biopsies were obtained at the beginning of the trial and at 1, 2 and 6 months.

They did not find any significant difference in the rate of cell proliferation between the calcium groups and the placebo group. On the other hand, when the daily calcium intake was increased via dairy foods the results were positive. These observations indicated the need for the studies that used dietary calcium for a longer period of time. Milk products may improve intestinal health by means of the intestinal cytoprotective effects of their high calcium phosphate content.

They proposed the following mechanism: the high amounts of colloidal calcium phosphate in milk products cause intestinal formation of insoluble, amorphous calcium phosphate (CaPi), which precipitates bile acids, fatty acids, and other unknown cytotoxic factors and thus inhibits colonic epithelial proliferation. Likewise, Glinghammer et al. found that a shift from a dairy product-free diet to a dairy product rich-diet, with a concomitant intake of milk protein and fat, did not change the genotoxicity of the colonic content but significantly reduced the cytotoxic compounds in the colon by precipitation.

It was also observed that these cytoprotective effects occurred throughout the intestine and therefore the mucosal damage was diminished and the resistance to an infection improved. There is considerable interest in the metabolic activities of the intestinal microflora in relation to the etiology of colon cancer. The human colon is intensively colonised with bacteria and as such an extremely complex microbial ecosystem. The majority of these residents are in fact benign and may even offer some health-promoting effect. The lactic acid bacteria termed probiotics are the most prominent representatives of the latter category.

Oral administration of certain probiotic bacteria is associated with a number of anticarcinogenic actions, including reduction of colonic pH, immunostimulation, anti-mutagenicity and reduction in the activity of enzymes responsible for the conversion of procarcinogens to carcinogens such as -glucuronidase, nitroreductase and azoreductase. Epidemiological studies have shown that consumption of fermented milk products, specially those containing probiotic bacteria, may help reduce the risk of cancer at a number of sites.

Milk proteins, especially those associated with whey, are most likely another milk components with anti-carcinogenic properties. Whey proteins are sulphur amino acids rich proteins and may therefore retard the development of colon tumors and tumor precursors through provision of biologically available methionine and cysteine. Both amino- acids have a positive influence on a cellular methylation status and therefore a stabilising effect on DNA. In addition, serum albumin, -lactalbumin and lactoferrin are rich sources of the dipeptide -glutamylcystein which is an excellent source of dietary cystein for cellular synthesis of glutathione an important actor in defence mechanisms that protect against cancer.

Whey also contains different high-affinity binding proteins that bind iron, folic acid, vitamin B_{12}, riboflavin, retinol and vitamin D. Their bioactivity is very important for keeping an organism in good healthy condition. Lactoferrin binds iron which is potentially pro-carcinogen and thus prevents intestinal damage, whereas the vitamin binding proteins protect vitamins from intestinal microflora as well as make them more bioavailable.

6

DIET, NUTRITION AND THE CHRONIC DISEASES

The diets people eat, in all their cultural variety, define to a large extent people's health, growth and development. Risk behaviours, such as tobacco use and physical inactivity, modify the result for better or worse. All this takes place in a social, cultural, political and economic environment that can aggravate the health of populations unless active measures are taken to make the environment a health-promoting one.

The rapidly increasing burden of chronic diseases is a key determinant of global public health. Already 79% of deaths attributable to chronic diseases are occurring in developing countries, predominantly in middleaged men. There is increasing evidence that chronic disease risks begin in fetal life and continue into old age (3–9). Adult chronic disease, therefore, reflects cumulative differential lifetime exposures to damaging physical and social environments.

For these reasons a life-course approach that captures both the cumulative risk and the many opportunities to intervene that this affords, was adopted by the Expert Consultation. While accepting the imperceptible progression from one life stage to the next, five stages were identified for convenience. **These are:** fetal development and the maternal environment; infancy; childhood and adolescence; adulthood; and ageing and older people.

FETAL DEVELOPMENT AND THE MATERNAL ENVIRONMENT

The four relevant factors in fetal life are:

a) Intrauterine growth retardation (IUGR);

b) Premature delivery of a normal growth for gestational age fetus;

c) Overnutrition in utero; and

d) Intergenerational factors.

There is considerable evidence, mostly from developed countries, that IUGR is associated with an increased risk of coronary heart disease, stroke, diabetes and raised blood pressure (9–20). It may rather be the pattern of growth, i. e. restricted fetal growth followed by very rapid postnatal catch-up growth, that is important in the underlying disease pathways. On the other hand, large size at birth (macrosomia) is also associated with an increased risk of diabetes and cardiovascular disease.

Among the adult population in India, an association was found between impaired glucose tolerance and high ponderal index (i. e. fatness) at birth. In Pima Indians, a U-shaped relationship to birth weight was found, whereas no such relationship was found amongst Mexican Americans. Higher birth weight has also been related to an increased risk of breast and other cancers. In sum, the evidence suggests that optimal birth weight and length distribution should be considered, not only in terms of immediate morbidity and mortality but also in regard to long-term outcomes such as susceptibility to diet-related chronic disease later in life.

Infancy Related Diseases

Retarded growth in infancy can be a reflected in a failure to gain weight and a failure to gain height. Both retarded growth and excessive weight or height gain ("crossing the centiles") can be factors in later incidence of chronic disease. An association between low growth in early infancy (low weight at 1 year) and an increased risk of coronary heart disease (CHD) has been described, irrespective of size at birth. Blood pressure has been found to be highest in those with retarded fetal growth and greater weight gain in infancy. Short stature, a reflection of socio-economic deprivation in childhood, is also associated with an increased risk of CHD and stroke, and to some extent, diabetes. The risk of stroke, and also of cancer mortality at several sites, including breast, uterus and colon, is increased if shorter children display an accelerated growth in height.

There is increasing evidence that among term and preterm infants, breast-feeding is associated with significantly lower blood pressure levels in childhood. Consumption of formula instead of breast milk in infancy has also been shown to increase diastolic and mean arterial blood pressure in later life. Nevertheless, studies with older cohorts and the Dutch study of famine have not identified such associations. There is increasingly strong evidence suggesting that a lower risk of developing obesity may be directly related to length of exclusive breast-feeding although it may not become evident until later in childhood.

Some of the discrepancy may be explained by socioeconomic and maternal education factors confounding the findings. Data from most, but not all, observational studies of term infants have generally suggested adverse effects of formula consumption on the other risk factors for cardiovascular disease (as well as blood pressure), but little information to support this finding is available from controlled clinical trials. Nevertheless, the weight of current evidence indicates adverse effects of formula milk on cardiovascular disease risk factors; this is consistent with the observations of increased mortality among older adults who were fed formula as infants.

The risk for several chronic diseases of childhood and adolescence (e. g. type 1 diabetes, coeliac disease, some childhood cancers, inflammatory bowel disease) have also been associated with infant feeding on breast-milk substitutes and short-term breast-feeding. There has been great interest in the possible effect of high-cholesterol feeding in early life. Reiser et. al. proposed the hypothesis that highcholesterol feeding in early life may serve to regulate cholesterol and lipoprotein metabolism in later life.

Animal data in support of this hypothesis are limited, but the idea of a possible metabolic imprinting served to trigger several retrospective and prospective studies in which cholesterol and lipoprotein metabolism in infants fed human milk were compared with those fed formula. Studies in suckling rats have suggested that the presence of cholesterol in the early diet may serve to define a metabolic pattern for lipoproteins and plasma cholesterol that could be of benefit later in life. The study by Mott, Lewis & McGill on differential diets in infant baboons, however, provided evidence to the contrary in terms of benefit.

Nevertheless, the observation of modified responses of adult cholesterol production rates, bile cholesterol saturation indices, and bile acid turnover, depending on whether the baboons were fed breast milk or formula, served to attract further interest. It was noted that increased atherosclerotic lesions associated with increased levels of plasma total cholesterol were related to increased dietary cholesterol in early life. No long-term human morbidity and mortality data supporting this notion have been reported. Short-term human studies have been in part confounded by diversity in solid food weaning regimens, as well as by the varied composition of fatty acid components of the early diet. The latter are now known to have an impact on circulating lipoprotein cholesterol species.

Mean plasma total cholesterol by age 4 months in infants fed breast milk reached 180 mg/dl or greater, while cholesterol values in infants fed formula tended to remain under 150 mg/dl. In a study by Carlson, DeVoe & Barness, infants receiving pre-dominantly a linoleic acidenriched oil blend exhibited a mean cholesterol concentration of approximately 110 mg/dl. A separate group of infants in that study who received pre-dominantly oleic acid had a mean cholesterol concentration of 133 mg/dl. Moreover, infants who were fed breast milk and oleic acid-enriched formula had higher high-density lipoprotein (HDL) cholesterol and apoproteins A-I and A-II than the pre-dominantly linoleic acid-enriched oil diet group.

The ratio of lowdensity lipoprotein (LDL) cholesterol plus very low-density lipoprotein (VLDL) cholesterol to HDL cholesterol was lowest for infants receiving the formula in which oleic acid was pre-dominant. Using a similar oleic acid pre-dominant formula, Darmady, Fosbrooke & Lloyd reported a mean value of 149 mg/dl at age 4 months, compared with 196 mg/dl in a parallel breast-fed group. Most of those infants then received an uncontrolled mixed diet and cow's milk, with no evident differences in plasma cholesterol levels by 12 months, independent of the type of early feeding they had received.

A more recent controlled study suggests that the specific fatty acid intake plays a pre-dominant role in determining total and LDL cholesterol. The significance of high dietary cholesterol associated with exclusive human milk feeding during the first 4 months of life has no demonstrated adverse effect. Measurements of serum lipoprotein concentrations and LDL receptor activity in infants suggests that it is the fatty acid content rather than the cholesterol in the diet which regulates cholesterol homeostasis. The regulation of endogenous cholesterol synthesis in infants appears to be regulated in a similar manner to that of adults.

Childhood and Adolescence Related Diseases

An association between low growth in childhood and an increased risk of CHD has been described, irrespective of size at birth. Although based only on developed country research at this point, this finding gives credence to the importance that is currently attached to the role of immediate postnatal factors in shaping disease risk. Growth rates in infants in Bangladesh, most of whom had chronic intrauterine undernourishment and were breastfed, were similar to growth rates of breastfed infants in industrialised countries, but catch-up growth was limited and weight at 12-months was largely a function of weight at birth.

In a study of 11–12 year-old Jamaican children, blood pressure levels were found to be highest in those with retarded fetal growth and greater weight gain between the ages of 7 and 11 years. Similar results were found in India. Low birth weight Indian babies have been described as having a characteristic poor muscle but high fat preservation, so-called "thin-fat" babies. This phenotype persists throughout the postnatal period and is associated with an increased central adiposity in childhood that is linked to the highest risk of raised blood pressure and disease. In most studies, the association between low birth weight and high blood pressure has been found to be particularly strong if adjusted to current body size – body mass index (BMI) – suggesting the importance of weight gain after birth.

Relative weight in adulthood and weight gain have been found to be associated with increased risk of cancer of the breast, colon, rectum, prostate and other sites. Whether there is an independent effect of childhood weight is difficult to determine, as childhood overweight is usually continued into adulthood. Relative weight in adolescence was significantly associated with colon cancer in one retrospective cohort study. Frankel, Gunnel & Peters, in the follow-up to an earlier survey by Boyd Orr in the late 1930s, found that for both sexes, after accounting for the confounding effects of social class, there was a significant positive relationship between childhood energy intake and adult cancer mortality.

The recent review by the International Agency for Research on Cancer (IARC) in Lyon, France, concluded that there was clear evidence of a relationship between onset of obesity (both early and later) and cancer risk. Short stature (including measures of childhood leg length), a reflection of socio-economic deprivation in childhood, is associated with an increased risk of CHD and stroke, and to some extent diabetes. Given that short stature, and specifically short leglength, are particularly sensitive indicators of early socio-economic deprivation, their association with later disease very likely reflects an association between early undernutrition and infectious disease load.

Height serves partly as an indicator of socio-economic and nutritional status in childhood. As has been seen, poor fetal development and poor growth during childhood have been associated with increased cardiovascular disease risk in adulthood, as have indicators of unfavourable social circumstances in childhood. Conversely, a high calorie intake in childhood may be related to an increased risk of cancer in later life. Height is inversely associated with mortality among men and women from all causes, including coronary heart disease, stroke and respiratory disease.

Height has also been used as a proxy for usual childhood energy intake, which is particularly related to body mass and the child's level of activity. However, it is clearly an imperfect proxy because when protein intake is adequate (energy appears to be important in this regard only in the first 3 months of life), genetics will define adult height. Protein, particularly animal protein, has been shown to have a selective effect in promoting height growth. It has been suggested that childhood obesity is related to excess protein intake and, of course, overweight or obese children tend to be in the upper percentiles for height.

Height has been shown to be related to cancer mortality at several sites, including breast, uterus and colon. The risk of stroke is increased by accelerated growth in height during childhood. As accelerated growth has been linked to development of hypertension in adult life, this may be the mechanism (plus an association with low socio-economic status). There is a higher prevalence of raised blood pressure not only in adults of low socio-economic status, but also in children from low socio-economic backgrounds, although the latter is not always associated with higher blood pressure later in life.

Blood pressure has been found to track from childhood to predict hypertension in adulthood, but with stronger tracking seen in older ages of childhood and in adolescence. High blood pressure in childhood (in combination with other risk factors) causes target organ and anatomical changes that are associated with cardiovascular risk, including reduction in artery elasticity, increased ventricular size and mass, haemodynamic increase in cardiac output and peripheral resistance. High blood pressure in children is strongly associated with obesity, in particular central obesity, and clusters and tracks with an adverse serum lipid profile (especially LDL cholesterol) and glucose intolerance.

There may be some ethnic differences, although these often seem to be explained by differences in body mass index. A retrospective mortality follow-up of a survey of family diet and health in the United Kingdom (1937–1939) identified significant associations between childhood energy intake and mortality from cancer. The presence and tracking of high blood pressure in children and adolescents occurs against a background of unhealthy lifestyles, including excessive intakes of total and saturated fats, cholesterol and salt, inadequate intakes of potassium, and reduced physical activity, often accompanied by high levels of television viewing.

In adolescents, habitual alcohol and tobacco use contributes to raised blood pressure. **There are three critical aspects of adolescence that have an impact on chronic diseases:**

a) The development of risk factors during this period;

b) The tracking of risk factors throughout life; and, in terms of prevention,

c) The development of healthy or unhealthy habits that tend to stay throughout life, for example physical inactivity because of television viewing.

In older children and adolescents, habitual alcohol and tobacco use contribute to raised blood pressure and the development of other risk factors in early life, most of which track into adulthood. The clustering of risk factor variables occurs as early as childhood and adolescence, and is associated with atherosclerosis in young adulthood and thus risk of later cardiovascular disease. This clustering has been described as the metabolic – or "syndrome X"

– clustering of physiological disturbances associated with insulin resistance, including hyperinsulinaemia, impaired glucose tolerance, hypertension, elevated plasma triglyceride and low HDL cholesterol. Raised serum cholesterol both in middle age and in early life are known to be associated with an increased risk of disease later on.

Serum cholesterol levels in adolescents and young white males were strongly related to subsequent risk of cardiovascular disease mortality and morbidity. Although the risk of obesity does not apparently increase in adults who were overweight at 1 and 3 years old, the risk rises steadily thereafter, regardless of parental weight. Tracking has also been reported in China, where overweight children were 2. 8 times as likely to become overweight adolescents; conversely, underweight children were 3. 6 times as likely to remain underweight as adolescents.

The study found that parental obesity and underweight, and the child's initial body mass index, dietary fat intake and family income helped predict tracking and changes. However, in a prospective cohort study conducted in the United Kingdom, little tracking from childhood overweight to adulthood obesity was found when using a measure of fatness (percentage body fat for age) that was independent of build. Only children obese at 13 years of age had an increased risk of obesity as adults, and that there was no excess adult health risk from childhood or adolescent overweight.

Interestingly, they found that in the thinnest children, the more obese they became as adults, the greater was their subsequent risk of developing chronic diseases. The real concern about these early manifestations of chronic disease, besides the fact that they are occurring earlier and earlier, is that once they have developed they tend to track in that individual throughout life. On the more positive side, there is evidence that they can be corrected. Overweight and obesity are, however, notoriously difficult to correct after becoming established, and there is an established risk of overweight during childhood persisting into adolescence and adulthood.

Recent analyses have shown that the later the weight gain in childhood and adolescence, the greater the persistence. More than 60% of overweight children have at least one additional risk factor for cardiovascular disease, such as raised blood pressure, hyperlipidaemia or hyperinsulinaemia, and more than 20% have two or more risk factors. Habits leading to noncommunicable disease development during adolescence It seems increasingly likely that there are widespread effects of early diet on later body composition, physiology and cognition. Such observations "provide strong support for the recent shift away from defining nutritional needs for prevention of acute deficiency symptoms towards long-term prevention of morbidity and mortality".

Increased birth weight increases the risk of obesity later, but children with low birth weight tend to remain small into adulthood. In industrialised countries there have been only modest increases in birth weight so the increased levels of obesity described earlier must reflect environmental changes. The "obesogenic" environment appears to be largely directed at the adolescent market, making healthy choices that much more difficult. At the same time, exercise patterns have changed and considerable parts of the day are spent sitting at school, in a factory, or in front of a television or computer.

Raised blood pressure, impaired glucose tolerance and dyslipidaemia are associated in children and adolescents with unhealthy lifestyles, such as diets containing excessive intakes of fats (especially saturated), cholesterol and salt, an inadequate intake of fibre and potassium, a lack of exercise, and increased television viewing.

Physical inactivity and smoking have been found independently to predict CHD and stroke in later life. It is increasingly recognised that unhealthy lifestyles do not just appear in adulthood but drive the early development of obesity, dyslipidaemia, high blood pressure, impaired glucose tolerance and associated disease risk. In many countries, changes in family eating patterns, including the increased consumption of fast foods, pre-prepared meals and carbonated drinks, have taken place over the past 30 years. At the same time, the amount of physical activity has been greatly reduced both at home and in school, as well as by increasing use of mechanised transport.

Adulthood Related Diseases

The three critical questions relating to adulthood were identified as:

a) To what extent do risk factors continue to be important in the development of chronic diseases;

b) To what extent will modifying such risk factors make a difference to the emergence of disease; and

c) What is the role of risk factor reduction and modification in secondary prevention and the treatment of those with disease?

Reviewing the evidence within the framework of a life-course approach highlights the importance of the adult phase of life, it being both the period during which most chronic diseases are expressed, as well as a critical time for the preventive reduction of risk factors and for increasing effective treatment. The most firmly established associations between cardiovascular disease or diabetes and factors in the lifespan are the ones between those diseases and the major known "adult" risk factors, such as tobacco use, obesity, physical inactivity, cholesterol, high blood pressure and alcohol consumption.

The factors that have been confirmed to lead to an increased risk of CHD, stroke and diabetes are: high blood pressure for CHD or stroke; high cholesterol (diet) for CHD, and tobacco use for CHD. Other associations are robust and consistent, although they have not necessarily been shown to be reversible: obesity and physical inactivity for CHD, diabetes and stroke; and heavy or binge drinking for CHD and stroke. Most of the studies are from developed countries, but supporting evidence from developing countries is beginning to emerge, for example, from India.

In developed countries, low socio-economic status is associated with higher risk of cardiovascular disease and diabetes. As in the affluent industrialised countries, there appears to be an initial preponderance of cardiovascular disease among the higher socio-economic groups, for example, as has been found in China. It is presumed that the disease will progressively shift to the more disadvantaged sectors of society. There is some evidence that this is already happening, especially among women in low-income groups, for example in Brazil and South Africa, as well as in countries in economic transition such as Morocco.

Other risk factors are continually being recognised or proposed. These include the role of high levels of homocysteine, the related factor of low folate, and the role of iron. From a social sciences perspective, Losier has suggested that socio-economic level is less important than a certain stability in the physical and social environment. In other words, an individual's sense of understanding of his or her environment, coupled with control over the course and setting of his or her own life appears to be the most important determinant of health. Marmot, among others, has demonstrated the impact of the wider environment and societal and individual stress on the development of chronic disease.

Diseases Affecting the Older People

There are three critical aspects relating to chronic diseases in the later part of the life-cycle:

a) Most chronic diseases will be manifested in this later stage of life;

b) There is an absolute benefit for ageing individuals and populations in changing risk factors and adopting health-promoting behaviours such as exercise and healthy diets; and

c) The need to maximize health by avoiding or delaying preventable disability.

Along with the societal and disease transitions, there has been a major demographic shift. Although older people are currently defined as those aged 60 years and above, this definition of older people has a very different meaning from the middle of the last century, when 60 years of age and above often exceeded the average life expectancy, especially in industrialised countries. It is worth remembering, however, that the majority of elderly people will, in fact, be living in the developing world. Most chronic diseases are present at this period of life – the result of interactions between multiple disease processes as well as more general losses in physiological functions. Cardiovascular disease peaks at this period, as does type 2 diabetes and some cancers. The main burden of chronic diseases is observed at this stage of life and, therefore, needs to be addressed.

In the 1970s, it was thought that risks were not significantly increased after certain late ages and that there would be no benefit in changing habits, such as dietary habits, after 80 years old as there was no epidemiological evidence that changing habits would affect mortality or even health conditions among older people. There was also a feeling that people "earned" some unhealthy behaviours simply because of reaching "old age". Then there was a more active intervention phase, when older people were encouraged to change their diets in ways that were probably overly rigorous for the expected benefit.

Morerecently, older people have been encouraged to eat a healthy diet – as large and as varied as possible while maintaining their weight – and particularly to continue exercise. Liu et al. have reported an observed risk of atherosclerotic disease among older women that was approximately 30% less in women who ate 5–10 servings of fruits and vegetables per day than in those who ate 2+5 servings per day. It seems that, as elderly patients have a higher cardiovascular risk, they are more likely to gain from risk factor modification.

Although this age group has received relatively little attention as regards primary prevention, the acceleration in decline caused by external factors is generally believed to be reversible at any age. Interventions aimed at supporting the individual and promoting healthier environments will often lead to increased independence in older age. Interactions between early and later factors throughout the life course Low birth weight, followed by subsequent adult obesity, has been shown to impart a particularly high risk of CHD, as well as diabetes. Risk of impaired glucose tolerance has been found to be highest in those who had low birth weight, but who subsequently became obese as adults.

A number of recent studies have demonstrated that there is an increased risk of adult disease when IUGR is followed by rapid catch-up growth in weight and height. Conversely, there is also fairly consistent evidence of higher risk of CHD, stroke, and probably adult onset diabetes with shorter stature. Further research is needed to define optimal growth in infancy in terms of prevention of chronic disease. A WHO multicentre growth reference study currently under way may serve to generate much needed information on this matter.

Impaired glucose tolerance and an adverse lipid profile are seen as early as childhood and adolescence, where they typically appear clustered together with higher blood pressure and relate strongly to obesity, in particular central obesity. Raised blood pressure, impaired glucose tolerance and dyslipidaemia also tend to be clustered in children and adolescents with unhealthy lifestyles and diets, such as those with excessive intakes of saturated fats, cholesterol and salt, and inadequate intake of fibre.

Lack of exercise and increased television viewing add to the risk. In older children and adolescents, habitual alcohol and tobacco use also contribute to raised blood pressure and to the development of other risk factors in early adulthood. Many of the same factors continue to act throughout the life course. Such clustering represents an opportunity to address more than one risk at a time. The clustering of health-related behaviours is also a well described phenomenon.

Young girls who grow poorly become stunted women and are more likely to give birth to low-birth-weight babies who are then likely to continue the cycle by being stunted in adulthood, and so on. Maternal birth size is a significant predictor of a child's birth size after controlling for gestational age, sex of the child, socio-economic status, and maternal age, height and pre-pregnant weight. There are clear indications of intergenerational factors in obesity, such as parental obesity, maternal gestational diabetes and maternal birth weight. Low maternal birth weight is associated with higher blood pressure levels in the offspring, independent of the relation between the offspring's own birth weight and blood pressure.

Unhealthy lifestyles can also have a direct effect on the health of the next generation, for example, smoking during pregnancy. There is good evidence that nutrients and physical activity influence gene expression and have shaped the genome over several million years of human evolution. Genes define opportunities for health and susceptibility to disease, while environmental factors determine which susceptible individuals will develop illness. In view of changing socio-economic conditions in developing countries, such added stress may result in exposure of underlying genetic predisposition to chronic diseases.

Gene-nutrient interactions also involve the environment. The dynamics of the relationships are becoming better understood but there is still a long way to go in this area, and also in other aspects, such as disease prevention and control. Studies continue on the role of nutrients in gene expression; for example, researchers are currently trying to understand why omega-3 fatty acids suppress or decrease the m-RNA of interleukin, which is elevated in atherosclerosis, arthritis and other autoimmune diseases, whereas the omega-6 fatty acids do not. Studies on genetic variability to dietary response indicate that specific genotypes raise cholesterol levels more than others.

The need for targeted diets for individuals and sub-groups to prevent chronic diseases was acknowledged as being part of an overall approach to prevention at the population level. However, the practical implications of this issue for public health policy have only begun to be addressed. For example, a recent study of the relationship between folate and cardiovascular disease revealed that acommonsingle gene mutation that reduces the activity of an enzyme involved in folate metabolism (MTHFR) is associated with a moderate (20%) increase in serum homocysteine and higher risk of both ischaemic heart disease and deep vein thrombosis.

Although humans have evolved being able to feed on a variety of foods and to adapt to them, certain genetic adaptations and limitations have occurred in relation to diet. Understanding the evolutionary aspects of diet and its composition might suggest a diet that would be consistent with the diet to which our genes were programmed to respond. However, the early diet was presumably one which gave evolutionary advantage to reproduction in the early part of life, and so may be less indicative of guidance for healthy eating, in terms of lifelong health and prevention of chronic disease after reproduction has been achieved.

Because there are genetic variations among individuals, changes in dietary patterns have a differential impact on a genetically heterogeneous population, although populations with a similar evolutionary background have more similar genotypes. There is a vast volume of scientific evidence highlighting the importance of applying a life-course approach to the prevention and control of chronic disease. The picture is, however, still not complete, and the evidence sometimes contradictory. **From the available evidence, it is possible to state the following:**

- Unhealthy diets, physical inactivity and smoking are confirmed risk behaviours for chronic diseases.
- The biological risk factors of hypertension, obesity and lipidaemia are firmly established as risk factors for coronary heart disease, stroke and diabetes.
- Nutrients and physical activity influence gene expression and may define susceptibility.
- The major biological and behavioural risk factors emerge and act in early life, and continue to have a negative impact throughout the life course.

- The major biological risk factors can continue to affect the health of the next generation.
- An adequate and appropriate postnatal nutritional environment is important.
- Globally, trends in the prevalence of many risk factors are upwards, especially those for obesity, physical inactivity and, in the developing world particularly, smoking.
- Selected interventions are effective but must extend beyond individual risk factors and continue throughout the life course.
- Some preventive interventions early in the life course offer lifelong benefits.
- Improving diets and increasing levels of physical activity in adults and older people will reduce chronic disease risks for death and disability.
- Secondary prevention through diet and physical activity is a complementary strategy in retarding the progression of existing chronic diseases and decreasing mortality and the disease burden from such diseases.

From the above, it is clear that risk factors must be addressed throughout the life course. As well as preventing chronic diseases, there are clearly many other reasons to improve the quality of life of people throughout their lifespan. The intention of primary prevention interventions is to move the profile of the whole population in a healthier direction. Small changes in risk factors in the majority who are at moderate risk can have an enormous impact in terms of population-attributable risk of death and disability.

By preventing disease in large populations, small reductions in blood pressure, blood cholesterol and so on can dramatically reduce health costs. For example, it has been demonstrated that improved lifestyles can reduce the risk of progression to diabetes by a striking 58% over 4 years. Other population studies have shown that up to 80% of cases of coronary heart disease, and up to 90% of cases of type 2 diabetes, could potentially be avoided through changing lifestyle factors, and about one-third of cancers could be avoided by eating healthily, maintaining normal weight and exercising throughout life.

For interventions to have a lasting effect on the risk factor prevalence and the health of societies, it is also essential to change or modify the environment in which these diseases develop. Changes in dietary patterns, the influence of advertising and the globalisation of diets, and widespread reduction in physical activity have generally had negative impacts in terms of risk factors, and presumably also in terms of subsequent disease. Reversing current trends will require a multifaceted public health policy approach.

While it is important to avoid inappropriately applying nutritional guidelines to populations that may differ genetically from those for whom the dietary and risk data were originally determined, to date the information regarding genes or gene combinations is insufficient to define specific dietary recommendations based on a population distribution of specific genetic polymorphisms. Guidelines should try to ensure that the overall benefit of recommendations to the majority of the population substantially outweighs any potential adverse effects on selected subgroups of the population. For example, population-wide efforts to prevent weight gain may trigger a fear of fatness and, therefore, undernutrition in adolescent girls.

The population nutrient goals recommended by the Joint WHO/FAO Expert Consultation at the present meeting are based on current scientific knowledge and evidence, and are intended to be further adapted and tailored to local or national diets and populations, where diet has evolved to be appropriate for the culture and local environment. The goals are intended to reverse or reduce the impact of unfavourable dietary changes that have occurred over the past century in the industrialised world and more recently in many developing countries.

Present nutrient intake goals also need to take into account the effects of long-term environmental changes, i. e. those that have occurred over time-scales of hundreds of years. For example, the metabolic response to periodic famine and chronic food shortage may no longer represent a selective advantage but instead may increase susceptibility to chronic diseases. An abundant stable food supply is a recent phenomenon; it was not a factor until the advent of the industrial revolution (or the equivalent process in more recently industrialised countries). A combination of physical activity, food variety and extensive social interaction is the most likely lifestyle profile to optimise health, as reflected in increased longevity and healthy ageing.

Some available evidence suggests that, within the time frame of a week, at least 20 and probably as many as 30 biologically distinct types of foods, with the emphasis on plant foods, are required for healthy diets. The current move towards increasing animal protein in diets in countries in economic transition is unlikely to be reversed in those countries where there are increased consumer resources, but is unlikely to be conducive to adult health, at least in terms of preventing chronic diseases. Finally, what success can be expected by developing and updating the scientific basis for national guidelines?

The percentage of British adults complying with national dietary guidelines is discouraging; for example, only 2–4% of the population are currently consuming the recommended level of saturated fat, and 5–25% are achieving the recommended levels of fibre. The figures would not be dissimilar in many other developed countries, where the majority of people are not aware of what exactly the dietary guidelines suggest.

7

GOALS FOR PREVENTING DIET-RELATED DISEASES

The population nutrient intake goals for consideration by national and regional bodies establishing dietary recommendations for the prevention of diet-related chronic diseases are presented below.

Total fat: The recommendations for total fat are formulated to include countries where the usual fat intake is typically above 30% as well as those where the usual intake may be very low, for example less than 15%. Total fat energy of at least 20% is consistent with good health. Highly active groups with diets rich in vegetables, legumes, fruits and wholegrain cereals may, however, sustain a total fat intake of up to 35% without the risk of unhealthy weight gain. For countries where the usual fat intake is between 15% and 20% of energy, there is no direct evidence for men that raising fat intake to 20% will be beneficial. For women of reproductive age at least 20% has been recommended by the Joint FAO/WHO Expert Consultation on Fats and Oils in Human Nutrition that met in 1993.

Free sugars: It is recognized that higher intakes of free sugars threaten the nutrient quality of diets by providing significant energy without specific nutrients.

The Consultation considered that restriction of free sugars was also likely to contribute to reducing the risk of unhealthy weight gain, **noting that:**

a) Free sugars contribute to the overall energy density of diets.

b) Free sugars promote a positive energy balance. Acute and short-term studies in human volunteers have demonstrated increased total energy intake when the energy density of the diet is increased, whether by free sugars or fat. Diets that are limited in free sugars have been shown to reduce total energy intake and induce weight loss.

c) Drinks that are rich in free sugars increase overall energy intake by reducing appetite control. There is thus less of a compensatory reduction of food intake after the consumption of high-sugars drinks than when additional foods of equivalent energy content are provided. A recent randomized trial showed that when soft drinks rich in free sugars are consumed there is a higher energy intake and a progressive increase in body weight when compared with energy-free drinks that are artificially sweetened. Children with a high consumption of soft drinks rich in free sugars are more likely to be overweight and to gain excess weight.

The Consultation recognized that a population goal for free sugars of less than 10% of total energy is controversial. However, the Consultation considered that the studies showing no effect of free sugars on excess weight have limitations. The CARMEN study (Carbohydrate Ratio Management in European National diets) was a multicentre, randomized trial that tested the effects on body weight and blood lipids in overweight individuals of altering the ratio of fat to carbohydrate, as well as the ratio of simple to complex carbohydrate per se. A greater weight reduction was observed with the high complex carbohydrate diet relative to the simple carbohydrate one; the difference, however was not statistically significant.

Nevertheless, an analysis of weight change and metabolic indices for those with metabolic syndrome revealed a clear benefit of replacing simple by complex carbohydrates. The Consultation also examined the results of studies that found an inverse relationship between free sugars intakes and total fat intake. Many of these studies are methodologically inappropriate for determining the causes of excess weight gain, since the percentage of calories from fat will decrease as the percentage of calories from carbohydrates increases and vice versa. Furthermore, these analyses do not usually distinguish between free sugars in foods and free sugars in drinks. Thus, these analyses are not good predictors of the responses in energy intake to a selective reduction in free sugars intake.

Non-starch polysaccharides (NSP): Whole grain cereals, fruits and vegetables are the preferred sources of non-starch polysaccharides (NSP). The best definition of dietary fibre remains to be established, given the potential health benefits of resistant starch. The recommended intake of fruits and vegetables and consumption of wholegrain foods is likely to provide >20 g per day of NSP (>25 g per day of total dietary fibre).

Fruits and vegetables: The benefit of fruits and vegetables cannot be ascribed to a single or mix of nutrients and bioactive substances. Therefore, this food category was included rather than the nutrients themselves. The category of tubers (i. e. potatoes, cassava) should not be included in fruits and vegetables.

Body mass index (BMI): For individuals, the recommendation is to maintain a BMI in the range 18.5

– 24.9 kg/m^2 and to avoid a weight gain greater than 5 kg during adult life.

Physical activity: The goal for physical activity focuses on maintaining healthy body weight. The recommendation is for a total of one hour per day on most days of the week of moderate-intensity activity, such as walking. This level of physical activity is needed to maintain a healthy body weight, particularly for people with sedentary occupations. The recommendation is based on calculations of energy balance and on an analysis of the extensive literature on the relationships between body weight and physical activity. This recommendation is also presented elsewhere. Obviously, this quantitative goal cannot be considered as a single "best value" by analogy with the nutrient intake goals.

In recommending physical activity, potential individual risks as well as benefits need to be assessed. In many regions of the world, especially but not exclusively in rural areas of developing countries, an appreciable proportion of the population is still engaged in physically demanding activities relating to agricultural practices and domestic tasks performed without mechanization or with rudimentary tools. Even children may be required to undertake physically demanding tasks at very young ages, such as collecting water and firewood and caring for livestock. Similarly, the inhabitants of poor urban areas may still be required to walk long distances to their jobs, which are usually of a manual nature and often require a high expenditure of energy. Clearly, the recommendation for extra physical activity is not relevant for these sectors of the population.

How to Prevent Diabetes

Measures aimed at reducing overweight and obesity, and cardiovascular disease are likely to also reduce the risk of developing type 2 diabetes and its complications. Some measures are particularly relevant to reducing the risk for diabetes; **these are listed below:**

- Prevention/treatment of overweight and obesity, particularly in highrisk groups.
- Maintaining an optimum BMI, i. e. at the lower end of the normal range. For the adult population, this means maintaining a mean BMI in the range 21–23 kg/m^2 and avoiding weight gain (>5 kg) in adult life.
- Voluntary weight reduction in overweight or obese individuals with impaired glucose tolerance (although screening for such individuals may not be cost-effective in many countries).
- Practising an endurance activity at moderate or greater level of intensity (e. g. brisk walking) for one hour or more per day on most days per week.
- Ensuring that saturated fat intake does not exceed 10% of total energy and for high-risk groups, fat intake should be <7% of total energy.
- Achieving adequate intakes of NSP through regular consumption of wholegrain cereals, legumes, fruits and vegetables. A minimum daily intake of 20 g is recommended.

How to Prevent Cardiovascular Diseases

The second half of the 20th century has witnessed major shifts in the pattern of disease, in addition to marked improvements in life expectancy, this period is characterized by profound changes in diet and lifestyles which in turn have contributed to an epidemic of non-communicable diseases. This epidemic is now emerging, and even accelerating, in most developing countries, while infections and nutritional deficiencies are receding as leading contributors to death and disability.

In developing countries, the effect of the nutrition transition and the concomitant rise in the prevalence of cardiovascular diseases will be to widen the mismatch between health care needs and resources, and already scarce resources will be stretched ever more thinly. Because unbalanced diets, obesity and physical inactivity all contribute to heart disease, addressing these, along with tobacco use, can help to stem the epidemic.

A large measure of success in this area has already been demonstrated in many industrialized countries. Cardiovascular diseases are the major contributor to the global burden of disease among the noncommunicable diseases. WHO currently attributes one-third of all global deaths (15.3 million) to CVD, with developing countries, low-income and middle-income countries accounting for 86% of the DALYs lost to CVD worldwide in 1998. In the next two decades the increasing burden of CVD will be borne mostly by developing countries. Measures aimed at reducing the risk of CVD are outlined below.

Fats: Dietary intake of fats strongly influences the risk of cardiovascular diseases such as coronary heart disease and stroke, through effects on blood lipids, thrombosis, blood pressure, arterial (endothelial) function, arrythmogenesis and inflammation. However, the qualitative composition of fats in the diet has a significant role to play in modifying this risk. EPA, eicosapentaenoic acid; DHA, docosahexaenoic acid; NSP, non-starch polysaccharides. The evidence shows that intake of saturated fatty acids is directly related to cardiovascular risk. The traditional target is to restrict the intake of saturated fatty acids to less than 10%, of daily energy intake and less than 7% for high-risk groups. If populations are consuming less than 10%, they should not increase that level of intake.

Within these limits, intake of foods rich in myristic and palmitic acids should be replaced by fats with a lower content of these particular fatty acids. In developing countries, however, where energy intake for some population groups may be inadequate, energy expenditure is high and body fat stores are low (BMI <18. 5 kg/m2). The amount and quality of fat supply has to be considered keeping in mind the need to meet energy requirements. Specific sources of saturated fat, such as coconut and palm oil, provide low-cost energy and may be an important source of energy for the poor. Not all saturated fats have similar metabolic effects; those with 12–16 carbons in the fatty acid chain have a greater effect on raising LDL cholesterol. This implies that the fatty acid composition of the fat source shouldbe examined.

As populations progress in the nutrition transitionand energy excess becomes a potential problem, restricting certain fatty acids becomes progressively more relevant to ensuring cardiovascular health. To promote cardiovascular health, diets should provide a very low intake of trans fatty acids (hydrogenated oils and fats). In practice, this implies an intake of less than 1% of daily energy intake. This recommendation is especially relevant in developing countries where low-cost hydrogenated fat is frequently consumed. The potential effect of human consumption of hydrogenated oils of unknown physiological effects (e. g. marine oils) is of great concern.

Diets should provide an adequate intake of PUFAs, i. e. in the range 6–10% of daily energy intake. There should also be an optimal balance between intake of n-6 PUFAs and n-3 PUFAs, i. e. 5–8% and 1–2% of daily energy intake, respectively. Intake of oleic acid, amonounsaturated fatty acid, should make up the rest of the daily energy intake from fats, to give a daily total fat intake ranging from 15% up to 30% of daily energy intake. Recommendations for total fat intake may be based on current levels of population consumption in different regions and modified to take account of age, activity and ideal body weight.

Where obesity is prevalent, for example, an intake in the lower part of the range is preferable in order to achieve a lower energy intake. While there is no evidence to directly link the quantity of daily fat intake to an increased risk of CVD, total fat consumption should be limited to enable the goals of reduced intake of saturated and trans fatty acids to be met easily in most populations and to avoid the potential problems of undesirable weight gain that may arise from unrestricted fat intake. It should be noted that highly active groups with diets rich in vegetables, legumes, fruits and wholegrain cereals will limit the risk of unhealthy weight gain on a diet comprising a total fat intake of up to 35%.

These dietary goals can be met by limiting the intake of fat from dairy and meat sources, avoiding the use of hydrogenated oils and fats in cooking and manufacture of food products, using appropriate edible vegetable oils in small amounts, and ensuring a regular intake of fish (one to two times per week) or plant sources of a-linolenic acid. Preference should be given to food preparation practices that employ non-frying methods.

Fruits and vegetables: Fruits and vegetables contribute to cardiovascular health through the variety of phytonutrients, potassium and fibre that they contain. Daily intake of fresh fruit and vegetables (including berries, green leafy and cruciferous vegetables and legumes), in an adequate quantity (400–500 g per day), is recommended to reduce the risk of coronary heart disease, stroke and high blood pressure.

Sodium: Dietary intake of sodium, from all sources,

influences blood pressure levels in populations and should be limited so as to reduce the risk of coronary heart disease and both forms of stroke. Current evidence suggests that an intake of no more than 70 mmol or 1.7 g of sodium per day is beneficial in reducing blood pressure. The special situation of individuals (i.e. pregnant women and non-acclimated people who perform strenuous physical activity in hot environments) who may be adversely affected by sodium reduction needs to be kept in mind.

Limitation of dietary sodium intake to meet these goals should be achieved by restricting daily salt (sodium chloride) intake to less than 5 g per day. This should take into account total sodium intake from all dietary sources, for example additives such as monosodium glutamate and preservatives. Use of potassium-enriched low-sodium substitutes is one way to reduce sodium intake. The need to adjust salt iodization, depending on observed sodium intake and surveillance of iodine status of the population, should be recognized.

Potassium: Adequate dietary intake of potassium lowers blood pressure and is protective against stroke and cardiac arrythmias. Potassium intake should be at a level which will keep the sodium to potassium ratio close to 1.0, i. e. a daily potassium intake level of 70–80 mmol per day. This may be achieved through adequate daily consumption of fruits and vegetables.

NSP (dietary fibre): Fibre is protective against coronary heart disease and has also been used in diets to lower blood pressure. Adequate intake may be achieved through fruits, vegetables and wholegrain cereals.

Fish: Regular fish consumption (1–2 servings per week) is protective against coronary heart disease and ischaemic stroke and is recommended. The serving should provide an equivalent of 200–500 mg of eicosapentaenoic and docosahexaenoic acid. People who are vegetarians are recommended to ensure adequate intake of plant sources of a-linolenic acid.

Alcohol: Although regular low to moderate consumption of alcohol is protective against coronary heart disease, other cardiovascular and health risks associated with alcohol do not favour a general recommendation for its use.

How to Prevent Cancer

Cancer is caused by a variety of identified and unidentified factors. The most important established cause of cancer is tobacco smoking. Other important determinants of cancer risk include diet, alcohol and physical activity, infections, hormonal factors and radiation. The relative importance of cancers as a cause of death is increasing, mostly because of the increasing proportion of people who are old, and also in part because of reductions in mortality from some other causes, especially infectious diseases.

The incidence of cancers of the lung, colon andrectum, breast and prostate generally increases in parallel with economic development, while the incidence of stomach cancer usually declines with development. Cancer is now a major cause of mortality throughout the world and, in the developed world, is generally exceeded only by cardiovascular diseases. An estimated 10 million new cases and over 6 million deaths from cancer occurred in 2000.

As developing countries become urbanized, patterns of cancer, including those most strongly associated with diet, tend to shift towards those of economically developed countries. Between 2000 and 2020, the total number of cases of cancer in the developing world is predicted to increase by 73% and, in the developed world, to increase by 29%, largely as a result of an increase in the number of old people.

The main recommendations for reducing the risk of developing cancer are as follows:

- Maintain weight (among adults) such that BMI is in the range of 18. 5–24. 9 kg/m^2 and avoid weight gain (>5 kg) during adult life.
- Maintain regular physical activity. The primary goal should be to perform physical activity on most days of the week; 60 minutes per day of moderate-intensity activity, such as walking, may be needed to maintain healthy body weight in otherwise sedentary people. More vigorous activity, such as fast walking, may give some additional benefits for cancer prevention.
- Consumption of alcoholic beverages is not recommended: if consumed, do not exceed two units1 per day.
- Chinese-style fermented salted fish should only be consumed in moderation, especially during childhood. Overall consumption of saltpreserved foods and salt should be moderate.
- Minimize exposure to aflatoxin in foods.
- Have a diet which includes at least 400 g per day of total fruits and vegetables.
- Those who are not vegetarian are advised to moderate consumption of preserved meat (e. g. sausages, salami, bacon, ham).
- Do not consume foods or drinks when they are at a very hot (scalding hot) temperature.

How to Prevent Dental Diseases

Oral health is related to diet in many ways, for

example, through nutritional influences on cranio-facial development, oral cancer and oral infectious diseases. The purpose of this review, however, is to focus on the nutritional aspects of dental diseases. Dental diseases include dental caries, developmental defects of enamel, dental erosion and periodontal disease. Dental diseases are a costly burden to health care services, accounting for between 5% and 10% of total health care expenditures and exceeding the cost of treating cardiovascular disease, cancer and osteoporosis in industrialized countries.

In low-income countries, the cost of traditional restorative treatment of dental disease would probably exceed the available resources for health care. Dental health promotion and preventive strategies are clearly more affordable and sustainable. Although not life-threatening, dental diseases have a detrimental effect on quality of life in childhood through to old age, having an impact on self-esteem, eating ability, nutrition and health.

In modern society, a significant role of teeth is to enhance appearance; facial appearance is very important in determining an individual's integration into society, and teeth also play an essential role in speech and communication. Oral diseases are associated with considerable pain, anxiety and impaired social functioning. Dental decay may result in tooth loss, which reduces the ability to eat a nutritious diet, the enjoyment of food, the confidence to socialize and the quality of life. Some specific recommendations are described below.

It is important to set a recommended maximum level for the consumption of free sugars; a low free sugars consumption by a population will translate into a low level of dental caries. Population goals enable the oral health risks of populations to be assessed and health promotion goals monitored. The best available evidence indicates that the level of dental caries is low in countries where the consumption of free sugars is below 15–20 kg per person per year. This is equivalent to a daily intake of 40–55 g per person and the values equate to 6–10% of energy intake.

It is of particular importance that countries which currently have low consumption of free sugars (<15–20 kg per person per year) do not increase consumption levels. For countries with high consumption levels it is recommended that national health authorities and decision-makers formulate country specific and community-specific goals for reduction in the amount of free sugars, aiming towards the recommended maximum of no more than 10% of energy intake.

In addition to population targets given in terms of the amount of free sugars, targets for the frequency of free sugars consumption are also important. The frequency of consumption of foods and/or drinks containing free sugars should be limited to a maximum of four times per day. Many countries that are currently undergoing nutrition transition do not have adequate exposure to fluoride. There should be promotion of adequate fluoride exposure via appropriate vehicles, for example, affordable toothpaste, water, salt and milk.

It is the responsibility of national health authorities to ensure implementation of feasible fluoride programmes for their country. In order to minimize the occurrence of dental erosion, the amount and frequency of intake of soft drinks and juices should be limited. Elimination of undernutrition prevents enamel hypoplasia and the other potential effects of undernutrition on oral health (e. g. salivary gland atrophy, periodontal disease, oral infectious diseases).

How to Prevent Osteoporosis

Osteoporosis is a disease affecting many millions of

people around the world. It is characterized by low bone mass and micro-architectural deterioration of bone tissue, leading to bone fragility and a consequent increase in risk of fracture. The incidence of vertebral and hip fractures increases exponentially with advancing age (while that of wrist fractures levels off after the age of 60 years). Osteoporosis fractures are a major cause of morbidity and disability in older people and, in the case of hip fractures, can lead to premature death. Such fractures impose a considerable economic burden on health services worldwide.

In countries with a high fracture incidence, a minimum of 400—500 mg of calcium intake is required to prevent osteoporosis. When consumption of dairy products is limited, other sources of calcium include fish with edible bones, tortillas processed with lime, green vegetables high in calcium (e. g. broccoli, kale), legumes and by-products of legumes (e. g. tofu). The interaction between calcium intake and physical activity, sun exposure, and intake of other dietary components (e. g. vitamin D, vitamin K, sodium, protein) and protective phytonutrients (e. g. soy compounds), needs to be considered before recommending increased calcium intake in countries with low fracture incidence in order to be in line with recommendations for industrialized countries.

With regard to calcium intakes to prevent osteoporosis, the Consultation referred to the recommendations of the Joint FAO/WHO Expert Consultation on Vitamin and Mineral Requirements in Human Nutrition which highlighted the calcium paradox. The paradox (that hip fracture rates are higher in developed countries where calcium intake is higher than in developing countries where calcium intake is lower) clearly calls for an explanation. To date, the accumulated data indicate that the adverse effect of protein, in particular animal (but not vegetable) protein, might outweigh the positive effect of calcium intake on calcium balance.

The report of the Joint FAO/WHO Expert Consultation on Vitamin and Mineral Requirements in Human Nutrition made it clear that the recommendations for calcium intakes were based on long-term (90 days) calcium balance data for adults derived from Australia, Canada, the European Union, the United Kingdom and the United States, and were not necessarily applicable to all countries worldwide.

The report also acknowledged that strong evidence was emerging that the requirements for calcium might vary from culture to culture for dietary, genetic, lifestyle and geographical reasons. Therefore, two sets of allowances were recommended: one for countries with low consumption of animal protein, and another based on data from North America and Western Europes. **The following conclusions were reached:**

a) There is no case for global, population-based approaches. A case can be made for targeted approaches with respect to calcium and vitamin D in high-risk sub-groups of populations, i. e. those with a high fracture incidence.

b) In countries with high osteoporotic fracture incidence, a low calcium intake (i. e. below 400–500 mg per day) among older men and women is associated with increased fracture risk.

c) In countries with high fracture incidence, increases in dietary vitamin D and calcium in the older populations can decrease fracture risk. Therefore, an adequate vitamin D status should be ensured. If vitamin D is obtained predominantly from dietary sources, for example, when sunshine exposure is limited, an intake of 5–10 mg per day is recommended.

d) Although firm evidence is lacking, prudent dietary and some lifestyle recommendations developed in respect of other chronic diseases may prove helpful in terms of reducing fracture risk. **These include:**

- increase physical activity;
- reduce sodium intake;
- increase consumption of fruits and vegetables;
- maintain a healthy body weight;
- avoid smoking;
- limit alcohol intake.

e) Convincing evidence indicates that physical activity, particularly activity that maintains or increases muscle strength, coordination and balance as important determinants of propensity for falling, is beneficial in prevention of osteoporotic fractures. In addition, regular lifetime weight-bearing activities, especially in modes that include impacts on bones and are done in vigorous fashion, increase peak bone mass in youth and help to maintain bone mass in later life.

8

CHILDREN AND FOOD ADVERTISING

The role of advertising and marketing food products to children and the extent to which it can be argued that such advertising makes a significant contribution to what the World Health Organisation (WHO) recognises as a serious health problem – obesity.

DIET

The concept of 'diet' seems as good a place as any as it seems central to the whole debate. The range of diets in the world and the structure and content of what is regarded as 'acceptable food' is vast, both historically and cross-culturally. The Southern Chinese regard dairy products such as cheese as inedible but many Europeans would find eating snake and dog unacceptable. Some cultures prefer food highly spiced and feed their children meat flavoured with, for the European palate, a ridiculous amount of chilli.

Indeed it seems to be the case that any and all combinations of animals, fruits and vegetables have appeared in the diet of some groups of people at some time in history. This rich variety of foods is not static and unchanging but alters over time, often over a matter of decades rather than centuries. In the UK, the preference for that great British dish, chicken tikka masala, is relatively recent.

And yet children start their dietary lives with just one source of food, which in many cases is the milk of their mother. There is a paradox here because most infants possess two characteristics that should predict a lack of change and development. They are notoriously neophobic where food is concerned, meaning that they dislike novelty and what has given satisfaction in the past will be selected in the future. The rewards of ingesting milk should then suggest a diet of warm, sticky, sweet fluids that produce a sleepy satiety. As well as that there is evidence that certain preferences, such as a liking for sugar, are built in and that we tend to seek out sugared foods.

The presence of clearly defined likes and dislikes at birth is adaptive since sweetness generally signals a safe source of carbohydrate, whereas sour and bitter tastes may signal danger. In studies of acceptance, infants preferentially consumed sugar solutions to water and even to formula. Newborn infants sugar solutions and photographed their reactions. The reaction to sweet tastes was one where many of the facial muscles relaxed, with a slight smile from the baby and often licking and sucking of the tongue. By contrast bitter and sour stimuli produced gaping or expulsive reactions in newborns.

There is also evidence that infants prefer foods with a high energy density as these produce a strong feeling of satiety after eating and these effects are more adaptive than low satiety. The innate preference for sweetness could be the end result of evolutionary pressure to ensure detection and recognition of food source that are likely to be high in calories. Rejection of bitterness and sourness may indicate a similar evolutionary pressure to avoid foods that are often inedible or even poisonous. So if children reject new foods and start off with a preference for sugared fluids and foods with a high energy density then how do we as adults end up with such a wide variety of foods and why do children adopt the dietary habits of their culture.

Fortunately from the point of view of gastronomy and for those who love food in all its different forms, children grow up as social animals and learn to change and adapt to cultural norms. From an early age children will model their food choices on the behaviour of the group, or on the behaviour of adults who consume other foods. So simple learning principles such as associative conditioning and modelling are enough to explain how new-born infants with their reliance on a single food source and an adaptive preference for high energy and sweet sources, can change after weaning to food consumption norms that are socially delivered by peers and family adults.

Pre-school children demonstrate an understanding of the cultural rules of diet. Acceptance for foods across the day in adults and children aged three to four years, as well as the appropriateness of a variety of foods for breakfast compared to dinner. Children demonstrated significant shifts in liking across the day and were clearly able to categorise food items according to their appropriateness for either breakfast or dinner.Thus even at three years of age, children are following cultural rules regarding appropriateness of foods for particular meals and therefore, young children are clearly able to recognise and implement culture-specific rules about foods.

The realm of food and food consumption, children are being influenced by two major agents of socialisation -family and friends. These two 'flesh and blood' social aspects of the child's existence are operative in the early childhood years and certainly before advertising is recognised by the child as such. Family and friends are also the most powerful agents of socialisation, including socialisation for preference and choice of different foods and diets. Media, and advertising, can be included as part of this, can influence children and we shall now look at just how this works.

NATURE OF FOOD ADVERTISING

If we look at 'what's on' in the sense of summarising just what foods are advertised to children then results are fairly consistent over the years. There has been a regular audit of US networks since the 1970s and the latest presents a picture that hasn't changed much. About two-thirds of the TV commercials on Saturday morning TV were for foods. Over half of these commercials were for breads, cereals, rice and pasta and the next largest category (28%) were fastfood outlets. The third major group was classified as 'fats, oils and sugars', which is a designated category used by the United States Department of Agriculture (USDA) if the primary ingredient by weight is either fat or sugar: there were 15% of these.

Now there is no reason to suppose that (a) taken together, the diet advertised on TV is portrayed as a balanced diet or (b) that if kids just ate what they saw then they would not be getting any fruit or vegetables, for example, as they are rarely (if ever) advertised. But it is often implicitly assumed that the more frequently children see a TV commercial for a branded food then they will proportionately consume more of that food. Consequently the foods advertised on TV and seen by the child should have a direct effect on the foods consumed by the child.

This is simply untrue and does not do justice to the complexity of food preference and choice and how advertising works within that framework. The reality is that food advertising to children is designed to increase or maintain the sales of a particular brand, rather than to increase the consumption of a particular category of food. Branding occurs in a competitive marketplace where the goods and services on offer are often very similar with regard to their instrumentality and functionality and need to be positioned in terms of their symbolic and expressive aspects.

The products on offer by one fast-food outlet are often very similar to another as they sell the same product. Branding can act as a handle on which to hang the differences between fast-food outlet X and fast-food outlet Y. Often the differences will be information about premium offers and tie-ins with other commercial partners, but they are also communicating information about status and image in order to establish a position in the constant jostling and manoeuvring that is part of today's global marketplace.

That is the reason why foods are advertised. In addition, foods such as sugared cereals that are frequently advertised to children are often bought by families, and the child has to negotiate within the family to get the brand into the shopping trolley and the mother will have the last word. Food advertising to children has an effect at the level of the brand and is operative against a backdrop of an already established set of food preferences and choices that is primarily determined by influences from the cultures of the family and peers.

There was no evidence that food advertising had an effect on the consumption of categories of food (such as foods high in fat or salt), although advertising might be successful in increasing brand consumption. There is no reason to change that statement in 2003. Having established that advertising has a role to play in children's food choice and preference but that there are various other more important factors operative, the next question is the role that food consumption habits and behaviours have in the development of obesity in children. The origins and extent of obesity in children today, it is important to establish one or two generally accepted facts about this condition.

OBESITY

The simplest definition of obesity is that it is the excessive accumulation of fat in the body. The cause of obesity is quite simple – fat accumulates when more calories are consumed than are expended. So this imbalance between calorie input and the corresponding expenditure of energy by exercise, for example, results over time in an accumulation of fat as adipose tissue. In order to ascertain the prevalence of obesity worldwide it is necessary to have an agreed measure.

In more general terms, what is the definition of body weight in relation to health outcomes. There are several ways of doing this and probably the best known is the body mass index (BMI). The formula for BMI is the individual's weight (in kilograms) divided by the square of their height (in metres). Normal BMIs are in the range 18.5-25 and we can set cut-off points of more than 30 as obesity, with 30-35 as moderate obesity, severe obesity as in the range 35-40, with anything above 40 classified as very severe obesity.

However BMI does not distinguish between weight associated with muscle and weight associated with fat, so that differences in body proportions and the relationship between BMI and body fat content can affect the BMI range considered to be outside the defined obese categories. These differences can be associated with groups that differ on, for example, sporting activity and also in terms of groups that are culturally and physically different.

Actuarial tables used by life assurance firms that relate mortality rates of men and women of different weights and heights are also used as other measures of being overweight or obese. These tables report 'typical' weight ranges for individuals of different heights, genders and frame sizes. Although there are different ways of measuring and classifying obesity in adults, it is more difficult to obtain valid indicators in children. However moves are advancing towards WHO approved measures, and BMI measures with age-related reference curves are available for a number of countries for both adults and children.

Nevertheless, BMI trends may have actually under-estimated the scale of the growth in obesity. BMI levels fell slightly during the 1980s before rising steeply in the 1990s and this probably reflected an initial shift of body mass from muscle to fat, with the loss of muscle masking the increase in fat. Waist circumference, which measures abdominal fat, has increased much more rapidly than BMI over the same period, implying an even steeper obesity trend. Measures of obesity are available and used extensively to obtain statistics on this problem worldwide. The measures are not without criticism, however, and results should be interpreted carefully.

Causes of Obesity

If we look at the causes of obesity then there is a general consensus that it is a multi-factorial problem; that is, there are many factors operating and they all interact with and mutually influence each other. There is absolutely no dis-agreement on that in the literature. It is important to emphasise that in multi-factorial situations the role of two or more factors can often be as a consequence of their interaction rather than a simple main effect of each taken separately.

Any genetic contribution to obesity will likely interact with environmental ones to produce a possible effect. Nevertheless, obesity is increasing and the WHO has claimed it is now pandemic. Twins were likely to be similar in body weight regardless of whether they were reared together or apart. The evidence for a genetic component exists and one writer has claimed that 'genetic factors are of overwhelming importance'. However, a genetic contribution does not mean that one's fate is predetermined by one's genes, and it is necessary for other factors to be in place before the genetic contribution is expressed.

The WHO considers 'that the genes involved in weight gain increase the risk or susceptibility of an individual to the development of obesity when exposed to an adverse environment'. The way this question is answered depends on the concept of heritability, which is an estimate, based on a statistical analysis of relevant data, that gives the proportion of influence provided by genes on a group of individuals. It is not a figure that suggests X% of one's behaviour is determined before one is born, and the previous comment about the interaction between environmental variables and any genetic contribution should be kept in mind.

Nevertheless, Bouchard claims that somewhere between 25% and 40% of the range of BMI indices in large samples can be attributed to heritability. The output side of the equation can be increased with exercise and the World Health Organisation states categorically that moderate physical activity is 'of profound significance' because the evidence suggests that there is a fundamental interaction between the level of physical activity and the proportion of dietary fat in determining whether energy balance can be sustained. People who sustain moderate or high levels of physical activity throughout life can tolerate diets with a high fat content (e.g. 35-40% of energy) whereas lower fat intakes (20-25% of energy) may be needed to minimise energy imbalance and weight gain in sedentary individuals and societies.

Obese women didn't eat more after exercise, and so did not compensate for the higher energy expenditure produced by exercise by increasing their intake. However, people who use cars and motorised transport and have sedentary leisure pursuits and work in an automated environment may find it difficult to achieve the required levels of physical activity simply by increasing their activity during 'leisure time'. Since this includes many of the inhabitants of a modern city, one would have to instigate regimes of regular and active physical activity from an early age such as walking and cycling to work and school.

The extent to which obesity is labelled as a problem is subject to cultural influence and often these cultural and sub-cultural values emerge from the economic activities of the society. In an important review of 144 published studies on socio-economic variations a pattern emerges where high socio-economic status (SES) is negatively correlated with obesity in developed countries for women. However, the reverse pattern is found in developing societies. For men, women, and children in developing societies there is a strong direct relationship between SES and obesity.

Sobal and Stunkard propose that the low prevalence of obesity in lower SES groups in developing societies could be a result of lack of food or even famine, coupled with high energy expenditure as a result of labour-intensive work patterns. Consequently the energy balance sheet is kept firmly in the red with little chance to accumulate a food 'income' with little expenditure of energy. With higher SES there is a greater opportunity to acquire food but there will also be cultural values favouring fat body shapes.

'Obesity may be a sign of health and wealth in developing societies, the opposite of its meaning in developed countries'. The history of peoples until very recently was often the history of food shortages and famines as harvests failed and rains didn't come. One is biologically predisposed to store and 'lay down' fat with great efficiency and in terms of the evolution of cultures it is not surprising that 'fatness' is a highly valued trait. Information available from 58-traditional cultures and 81% of them considered 'plumpness' an ideal of feminine beauty. For example, in Nigeria pubescent daughters of the wealthy are sent to 'fattening huts' before marriage.

Together with social mobility in developing countries it is possible to find malnutrition and obesity coexisting in the same setting, as Peña and Bacallao found recorded in Brazil in the distribution of anthropometric data including BMI indices. In industrialised and developed countries on the other hand, obesity is a severely stigmatised condition among women but not with men.

Women from girlhood through adolescence to adulthood are quite willing to accept the stigma, although there is a critique that challenges assumptions of thinness in women. British longitudinal studies have shown that SES of origin is almost as strongly related to the prevalence of obesity and thinness as the adult's own SES, showing that the circumstances and values of life in the socio-economic class into which one is born may transmit pressures for thinness to adolescent girls during their socialisation. 'The more a woman believes that what is fat is bad, that what is thin is beautiful, and beautiful is good, the more she will work toward thinness and be distressed about fatness'.

So in general there is a constellation of environmental,

social, economic, psychological, and genetic factors that constitute a multi-factorial mix contributing to obesity. The (rather awkward) term 'obesogenic' has been coined to describe the cultural and environmental 'style' that is conducive towards an imbalance in energy input/output, promoting obesity.

It refers to an environment in which fertility rates are falling, life expectancy is growing, social structures are changing the family dramatically and urban development is growing, children have fewer safe places to play, there is declining agriculture, an increase in working mothers and less home-cooked food. All of these taken together are conducive to the development of obesity globally. This environment, it is claimed, promotes sedentary lifestyles and altered dietary habits.

In 2000, the World Health Organisation (WHO) produced a report that warned governments about a growing epidemic that threatened public health: obesity. In some countries gave a warning that obesity could soon kill as many people each year as cigarette-smoking. The World Health Organisation (WHO) general assembly, held in May 2004 in Geneva, had on its agenda a document entitled 'World Strategy for Food, Physical Exercise and Health'. In addition to information and awareness campaigns, the WHO recommended a more stringent regulation on advertisement and labelling of foodstuffs, because 'consumers have the right to obtain correct, standardised and understandable information on the contents of foodstuffs, so as to make enlightened choices'.

The WHO's forecasts predicted that cardiovascular diseases would be the first cause of mortality in developing countries by 2010, a status that is already the case in the industrialised countries. Atherosclerosis – a disease associated with the consumption of foods containing too much fat and sugars, a sedentary lifestyle and smoking together with type-2 diabetes and obesity are real world epidemics. The increase in the number of persons suffering from type-2 diabetes is a matter of high concern.

The figure of 150 million patients may double in 2005 especially with the rise of those in pre-diabetic stages, characterised by intolerance to glucose and abnormal glycaemia before breakfast, as well as in the frequency of the metabolic syndrome. The latter is probably three to four times more frequent than the established type-2 diabetes, and it is a combination of obesity (specially an excess of abdominal fat, with an increase of girth), an abnormal content of lipids (particularly triglycerides) in the blood, and hypertension. This syndrome is caused by an excess of body fat, especially in the abdomen, a sedentary way of life and inappropriate eating habits.

In addition, the release of great quantities of free fatty acids by the body fatty tissue results in insulin resistance; as the activity of the hormone is inhibited, glucose cannot penetrate into the muscles and consequently glycaemia rises. There is also the release by the fatty tissue of adipocytokines, anti-inflammatory substances that reduce the secretion of another hormone, adiponectin, which normally protects against insulin resistance and inflammation. Being overweight increases the risk of suffering from several related illnesses and may contribute to an earlier death. Women who are overweight run a risk five times higher than average of developing type-2 diabetes while those who are severely obese have a risk of more than 50 times higher.

Obesity is also implicated in cancer: A recent study in USA showed that 14 per cent of cancer deaths in men and 20 per cent in women could be attributed to it. Being overweight is also one of the main causes of heart diseases, the world's major cause of death, above wars, malaria and AIDS. This problem does not seem less acute in the developing world. Asians and black Africans are even more susceptible to obesity and its related diseases than are Caucasians. For instance, 3 per cent of Chinese and 5.5 per cent of Indians are diabetic, compared with 3 per cent of British people.

There are more new cases of diabetes in China and India than there are in the rest of the world put together. This is despite the fact that China was already spending 1.6 per cent of its annual gross domestic product treating non-communicable diseases, mostly obesity-related. The finger of blame seems to point to eating habits and also at the quality of foodstuffs (with implications for food manufacturing companies). The trend in food manufacturing has been to produce cheaper food, which in some ways could have adverse human health effects.

For instance, hydrogenated vegetable oil – vegetable fat made solid by adding hydrogen atoms – is the nutritionists' current enemy. Widely used as a cheap substitute for butter and cream, it is the main dietary source of trans-fatty acids, heavily implicated in heart diseases. Some companies are therefore removing them from their products for fear of lawsuits. Cheap food may also make people eat more, and food companies certainly think giving people more food for their money makes them buy more. That is why portions of manufactured food and soft drinks have been growing in size and volume. Companies are now increasingly under pressure to stop selling to people more food for less money, but it is hard to reverse that trend.

Tasty foodstuffs are generally sugary, fatty and salty. Taste is as much instinct as habit, and once people are used to sugary, fatty and salty foods, they find it hard to give them up. Producing healthier foodstuffs that are also attractive to consumers' tastes could help solve the problem, in addition to education on better nutrition, food consumption habits and regular exercise. Health food is not a turn-of-the-21st-century invention.

In 1985, people gave up caffeine; in 1987, salt; in 1994, fat. Now it is carbohydrates. But contemporary health-food consciousness may have stronger foundations. The need for healthier food may also be a matter of demographics across timelines related to "demographic evolution" as the president of food system design at Cargill, Inc., pointed out. In 1975, there were 230 million over 65 years of age; 420 million in 2000 and 830 million was the estimate for 2025. As people become older, their willingness to spend money on staying healthy increases.

Science has also contributed to the growing healthy-food consciousness. According to New Nutrition Business, a US consultancy firm, in 1996 there were 120 papers on nutrition science in peer-reviewed journals; in 2002, there were over 1000. With more scientific data, regulators (in the USA at least) are more willing to evaluate products and if so found with basis, allow health claims on products; and health claims increase sales. The At kins diet, during its peak days, which has boosted sales of eggs and meat, and hit potatoes, is one manifestation of consumers' determination to try various ways of programming their eating habits.

Supermarkets also cater to this market. For instance, Waitrose's Perfectly Balanced Meals claim no more than 4 per cent fat, very little salt and no 'butylated hydroxanisole or hydroxytoluene' at all; and sales are rising at 20-25 per cent annually. Sales of nutritional supplements have more than doubled in the USA in the six years after the Food and Drug Administration (FDA) liberalised labelling laws. In 2000, sales amounted to Rs. 765 billion and were increasing at 10 per cent a year.

In the United Kingdom, by the end of February 2004, a report on public health commissioned by the government cited obesity among its main worries. Previous to that, the Prime Minister's strategy unit floated the idea of a 'fat- tax' on foods that induce obesity; and in 2003, the Food Standards Agency – the industry regulation – advocated a ban on advertising junk food to children. Yet the UK government dismissed the idea of a fat tax, and the culture secretary stated she was skeptical about an advertising ban. The health secretary said the government wanted to be neither a 'nanny state' nor a 'Pontius Pilate state, which washes its hands of its citizens' health'.

Obesity among children

In France, obesity among children has been increasing since the early 1970s, particularly in the least-privileged social categories. The percentage of overweight schoolchildren has increased from 3 percent in 1965 to 5 percent in 1980, 12 percent in 1996 and 16 percent in 2003. The current figures are those prevailing in the USA during the 1970s, but the rate of increase is similar to that of the US. This illness has become a major challenge to public health and has been considered an epidemic by the French National Institute for Health and Medical Research (INSERM).

According to Jean-Philippe Ginardet of the Trousseau hospital in Paris, obesity among children is a frequent, serious and societal disease, difficult to treat, which leads, in the short term, to hypertension, diabetes and increase in the concentration of blood cholesterol. It paves the way for cardiovascular diseases among adults, i.e. for the first cause of mortality. Since 1992, evaluations have been carried out in schools of two cities in northern France. The first evaluation showed that children informed by their teachers had better nutritional knowledge and could therefore adopt better eating habits. The second evaluation, carried out in 1992 and 1997, revealed that within the families substantial change had occurred with respect to a better schedule of meals and to a significant reduction of animal fats in their diet.

As a result, between 1997 and 2000, the incidence of obesity in the children in these cities has increased much less: +4 percent among girls and +1 percent among boys compared to the whole region (Nord-Pas-de-Calais) that showed an increase of 95 percent among girls and +195 per cent among boys. This experimental approach to preventing obesity has lead to the launching of a five-year campaign named 'Together, let us prevent obesity among children' by the Observatory of Food Habits and Weight, and the Association for the Prevention and Treatment of Obesity in Pediatrics.

Obesity is not a disease that is treated only with the assistance of physicians; it also concerns the family and society as a whole. While there may be basis to claim that the lack of exercise and the increasing time spent watching the television or using the computer, as well as junk food are considered important causal factors, obesity's etiology is not confined to lifestyles and habits. Family histories play an important role too, supported by the fact that 57- percent of obese children have at least one overweight parent. This underlines the genetic role as well as the conditions attending to the pre- and post-natal periods and to subsequent psychic and social factors in causing obesity.

New epidemiological studies are needed to better understand the causes of the obesity epidemic. In France, a number of measures have been taken by the Ministry of Health within the framework of their National Programme for Nutrition Health (PNNS), launched in 2001 and the nine priority objectives which aim at stopping the prevalence of obesity among children. These include: the distribution of food and education activities in some primary and secondary schools; setting up a working group on 'food- advertisement and the child' with a view to reaching a compromise between the economic interests of the agri-food industry and public health constraints; recommendations to support breastfeeding; publication of a guide for children and teenagers on food and nutrition.

Physicians are requested to detect obesity as early as possible on the basis of reference graphs and a disk for measuring the index of body mass provided to them since November 2003. The WHO guide to measuring this index is as follows: the ratio of body weight (in kg) to height (in meters) raised to the power of 2; a resulting number above 25 is considered overweight and above 30 is "obese." These tools enable the physician to find out the period within which the accumulation of fat occurs – whether it is between the ages of 5-6 years and or before. With only a 38% success rate of treatment among children, early detection of obesity may improve their chances.

In Italy, since the early 1990s a centre has been working on the treatment of obesity among children in Atri, a small town of 11,000 inhabitants in the Abruzzes region. A recent survey in elementary schools showed that 31.6 percent of children had a weight above the norm and 6.7 percent of them were obese. Of the latter, the centre's physicians considered that only 5 percent of obesity cases could be related to genetic or endocrine causes, while the rest were caused by bad eating habits. It did not seem to be a question of quantity of food but of poor eating habits.

Among these habits the physicians listed: the lack of breakfast, too many snacks composed of industrial foodstuffs, lack of, or very little consumption of fresh fruit and vegetables. The absence of exercise was also an aggravating factor. The treatment of obesity cases begins with the involvement of the family. Once a week, children should come to the centre with their parents and sometimes with their grandparents (if the latter are those who cook at home). In the centre's restaurant, a meal is served to them, containing pasta without fat, fish, fruit and vegetables.

Children are not forced to eat meals to which they are not accustomed; they just have to try. The parents also eat the same meals. Then the children meet with the psychologist and nutritionist; the parents follow. Family participation is crucial, because the parents should familiarise themselves with the carefully prepared and measured meals and above all they must understand that the children should not eat quickly, that pasta should not be left aside, that they should not eat while watching television, because this usually causes the child to lose control of what he/she eats.

The whole family should re-consider its way of preparing meals and eating them; that is why the centre's specialists insist that both children and grown-ups have their meals together and eat the same foodstuffs. During the summer, about 40 children between 7 and 10 years old are welcomed in a camp, located in a rural tourist centre seven kilometers from Atri. At the summer camp, children's nutrition is strictly controlled and physical exercise is a frequent practice, while television is prohibited. The objective is to consolidate the new relationship between children and their food. They learn how to identify foodstuffs through blind-tasting, i.e., they develop their sense of smell and touch through handling them. It has been observed that children who attend the summer camp make remarkable progress with respect to their nutritional health and eating habits.

Changing Eating Habits

People are consuming more and more food outside their homes. They eat in bars, restaurants, and other catering enterprises. The latest figures on the consumer barometer indicated that confidence in foodstuffs was undergoing a slow but sustained increase, in the European Union, with the notable exception of fast food. In the Mediterranean countries, the onslaught of fast food has destroyed good feeding habits but instead of the expected high obesity rate, the Mediterranean diet resulted in less cholesterol in the blood, and higher life expectancy. But a study by Eurostat – the Statistics Centre of the European Union warned that the South was no longer what it was.

Not only have the Latins ceased to be slimmer than the Germans and the British. No less than 34.4 percent of Greek men were overweight, as opposed to 29.5 percent of their British counterparts and 28 percent of Germans. The Greek population now possesses the highest proportion of overweight members among countries of the European Union, followed by Spain with 32%. However, the Greeks had the lowest rate of dementia among the over 65's, and they still enjoy one of the highest life expectancies in the EU, with outstanding defenses against colon cancer, hypertension and heart attacks. This maybe attributed to their high consumption rates for olive oil – 20 litres per person per annum – i.e. seven times more than the Spaniards'.

Some years ago, attention was drawn to the 'Mediterranean paradox': Spain, France and Italy had fewer cardiovascular illnesses than their neighbours in Northern Europe, even though there were no significant differences in body weight. The difference lay in the diet, which includes abundant fruit and vegetables (rich in vitamins and antioxidants), olive oil as the main source of fat (as opposed to an excessive use of butter and other saturated fats), more fish (rich in omega-3 fatty acids which protect blood vessels), the reasonable consumption of wine with meals (one glass a day has an anti-oxidant effect and may increase the content of high-density lipoproteins – HDL– in the blood), and of generous inclusions of garlic, onions and nuts.

However, in time, the greater consumption of meat and lesser consumption of vegetables, more sauces rather than oil and vinegar dressings, whisky and other spirits instead of wine, soft drinks instead of water, and a sedentary lifestyle have led to more digestive problems, higher blood pressure and more kidney failures and respiratory illnesses. According to the Spanish sociologist and journalist Vicente- Verdú, 'health has declined proportionally with the rise in the economy, and gastronomic ignorance has spread in pace with the cultural revolution.

In the United Kingdom, there were signs that the problem of obesity was not necessarily worsening. For instance, while it enjoys the title of being one of the world's biggest consumers of chocolate, over the four years to 2002, sales of chocolate fell every year: 2 percent by volume and 7 percent by value over the period. In February 2004, the new chief executive officer of Nestlé Rowntree described it as 'a business in crisis'; although the company denied later on that there was a crisis, admitting only that sales of Kit Kat, its widely-known brand, fell by 2 percent in 2003.

Cadbury Schweppes, the United Kingdom's biggest producer of fattening foodstuffs, stated that five years ago, chocolate made it up to 80 per cent of sales; that was now down to a half. Five years ago, 85 percent of sold beverages were sweet; that is now down to 56 percent. The rest was mostly juice. Sale of diet drinks – which made up a third of the sales of fizzy drinks – have been growing at 5 percent a year, while sales of fattening foodstuffs had been stagnant. In British supermarkets, people are buying healthier food.

According to Tesco's director of corporate affairs, its

Healthy Living (lower calorie) range grew by 12 percent in 2003, twice the growth in overall sales. Sales of fruit and vegetables were growing faster than overall sales, too. That may be partly because fresh produce is becoming more varied, there are more of them available all year round and better supply encourages more demand. Five years ago, Tesco stocked six or seven varieties of tomato, while nowadays it stocks 15.

A study carried out by the University of Southampton on a big new supermarket in a poor area of Leeds concluded that after it opened, two-thirds of those with the worst diets now ate more fruit and vegetables. Cafes and restaurants report an increase in healthy eating too. Prêt-A-Manger, a sandwich chain, stated that sales of salads grew by 63 per cent in 2003, compared with 6 percent overall sales growth. Even McDonald's, which introduced fruit salad by early 2003, had sold 10 million portions since.

There are also good signs in the area of physical exercise. Gym membership figures suggest that British people at least intend to be less indolent. According to Mintel, a market-research company, there were 3.8 million members of private gyms in 2003, up from 2.2 million in 1998. The overall results of these favourable trends was that the average man became thinner in 2002 while women's BMI was static, at least according to body-mass-index (BMI) which have only began to be recorded in 2002. One year of course does not make a trend, but a decrease in America's weight in 2003, also for the first time, supports the idea that something is changing in the obesity trends of the two of the most developed countries in the world.

On the other hand, where the rich lead, the poor tend to follow – partly because the poor become richer over time, and partly because health messages tend to reach the better-educated first and the less-educated later. That happened with smoking, which the rich countries gave up years ago, and the poor are nowadays trying to abandon. As for government intervention in reducing obesity rates, campaigners for the "fat tax" point out that that this kind of intervention could aid the efforts to reduce obesity rates as government intervention did for smoking.

But that may not necessarily be the case with food because consumers now are constantly assailed by messages from companies telling them to lose weight. Also, peer pressure among teens on weight issues may have more impact on teenagers than ministerial action. However, some forms of government intervention have triumphed. For example, on 8 April 2004, the French parliament examined a bill that aimed at prohibiting automatic machines vending confectionery and soda in schools, and also on setting new rules on the advertisement of foodstuffs during television shows targeted to youth.

On 30 July 2004, the French Parliament voted in favour of prohibiting as of 1 September 2005 vending machines in schools. This vote was cheered by 250 pediatricians and nutritionists working in hospitals who earlier on wrote to the minister of health a letter titled 'For a consistent nutrition policy of public health in France'. The French traditional morning snack has been questioned. In January 2004, the French Agency for Food Sanitary Safety (AFSSA) has published an advice against it; the Agency stated that the concern about compensating food insufficiency among a small minority of children (less than 10 per cent attend school without having had breakfast) leads to an unbalance of the diet of all schoolchildren; the additional food intake causes an excess of calories which leads to an increase in the obesity rate among children.

ETIOLOGICAL FACTORS

The potential etiological factors related to unhealthy weight gain are listed below.

Convincing Etiological Factors

Regular physical activity (protective) and sedentary lifestyles (causative): There is convincing evidence that regular physical activity is protective against unhealthy weight gain whereas sedentary lifestyles, particularly sedentary occupations and inactive recreation such as watching television, promote it. Most epidemiological studies show smaller risk of weight gain, overweight and obesity among persons who currently engage regularly in moderate to large amounts of physical activity. Studies measuring physical activity at baseline and randomised trials of exercise programmes show more mixed results, probably because of the low adherence to long-term changes.

Therefore, it is ongoing physical activity itself rather than previous physical activity or enrolment in an exercise programme that is protective against unhealthy weight gain. The recommendation for individuals to accumulate at least 30 minutes of moderate-intensity physical activity on most days is largely aimed at reducing cardiovascular diseases and overall mortality. The amount needed to prevent unhealthy weight gain is uncertain but is probably significantly greater than this. Preventing weight gain after substantial weight loss probably requires about 60–90 minutes per day.

Two meetings recommended by consensus that about 45–60 minutes of moderate-intensity physical activity is needed on most days or every day to prevent unhealthy weight gain. Studies aimed at reducing sedentary behaviours have focused primarily on reducing television viewing in children. Reducing viewing times by about 30 minutes a day in children in the United States appears feasible and is associated with reductions in BMI.

A high dietary intake of non-starch polysaccharides (NSP)/dietary fibre (protective): The nomenclature and definitions of NSP (dietary fibre) have changed with time, and many of the available studies used previous definitions, such as soluble and insoluble fibre. Nevertheless, two recent reviews of randomised trials have concluded that the majority of studies show that a high intake of NSP (dietary fibre) promotes weight loss. Pereira & Ludwig found that 12 out of 19 trials showed beneficial objective effects (including weight loss). In their review of 11 studies of more than 4 weeks duration, involving ad libitum eating Howarth Saltzman & Roberts reported a mean weight loss of 1. 9 kg over 3. 8 months. There were no differences between fibre type or between fibre consumed in food or as supplements.

High intake of energy-dense micronutrient-poor foods (causative). There is convincing evidence that a high intake of energy-dense foods promotes weight gain. In high-income countries (and increasingly in lowincome countries) these energy-dense foods are not only highly processed (low NSP) but also micronutrient-poor, further diminishing their nutritional value. Energy-dense foods tend to be high in fat (e. g. butter, oils, fried foods), sugars or starch, while energy-dilute foods have a high water content (e. g. fruits and vegetables). Several trials have covertly manipulated the fat content and the energy density of diets, the results of which support the view that so-called "passive over consumption" of total energy occurs when the energy density of the diet is high and that this is almost always the case in high-fat diets.

A meta-analysis of 16 trials of ad libitum high-fat versus low-fat diets of at least 2 months duration suggested that a reduction in fat content by 10% corresponds to about a 1 MJ reduction in energy intake and about 3 kg in body weight. At a population level, 3 kg equates to about one BMI unit or about a 5% difference in obesity prevalence. However, it is difficult to blind such studies and other non-physiological effects may influence these findings. While energy from fat is no more fattening than the same amount of energy from carbohydrate or protein, diets that are high in fat tend to be energy-dense.

An important exception to this is diets based predominantly on energy-dilute foods (e. g. vegetables, legumes, fruits) but which have a reasonably high percentage of energy as fat from added oils. The effectiveness over the long-term of most dietary strategies for weight loss, including low-fat diets, remains uncertain unless accompanied by changes in behaviour affecting physical activity and food habits. These latter changes at a public health level require an environment supportive of healthy food choices and an active life. High quality trials to address these issues are urgently needed.

A variety of popular weight-loss diets that restrict food choices may result in reduced energy intake and short-term weight loss in individuals but most do not have trial evidence of long-term effectiveness and nutritional adequacy and therefore cannot be recommended for populations.

Probable Etiological Factors

Home and school environments that promote healthy food and activity choices for children (protective): Despite the obvious importance of the roles that parents and home environments play on children's eating and physical activity behaviours, there is very little hard evidence available to support this view. It appears that access and exposure to a range of fruits and vegetables in the home is important for the development of preferences for these foods and that parental knowledge, attitudes and behaviours related to healthy diet and physical activity are important in creating role models.

More data are available on the impact of the school environment on nutrition knowledge, on eating patterns and physical activity at school, and on sedentary behaviours at home. Some studies, but not all, have shown an effect of school-based interventions on obesity prevention. While more research is clearly needed to increase the evidence base in both these areas, supportive home and school environments were rated as a probable etiological influence on obesity.

Heavy marketing of fast-food outlets and energy-dense, micronutrientpoor foods and beverages (causative): Part of the consistent, strong relationships between television viewing and obesity in children may relate to the food advertising to which they are exposed. Fastfood restaurants, and foods and beverages that are usually classified under the "eat least" category in dietary guidelines are among the most heavily marketed products, especially on television.

Young children are often the target group for the advertising of these products because they have a significant influence on the foods bought by parents. The huge expenditure on marketing fast-foods and other "eat least" choices was considered to be a key factor in the increased consumption of food prepared outside the home in general and of energy-dense, micronutrient-poor foods in particular.

Young children are unable to distinguish programme content from the persuasive intent of advertisements. The evidence that the heavy marketing of these foods and beverages to young children causes obesity is not unequivocal. Nevertheless, the Consultation considered that there is sufficient indirect evidence to warrant this practice being placed in the "probable" category and thus becoming a potential target for interventions.

A high intake of sugars-sweetened beverages (causative): Diets that are proportionally low in fat will be proportionally higher in carbohydrate (including a variable amount of sugars) and are associated with protection against unhealthy weight gain, although a high intake of free sugars in beverages probably promotes weight gain. The physiological effects of energy intake on satiation and satiety appear to be quite different for energy in solid foods as opposed to energy in fluids. Possibly because of reduced gastric distension and faster transit times, the energy contained in fluids is less well "detected" by the body and subsequent food intake is poorly adjusted to account for the energy taken in through beverages. This is supported by data from cross-sectional, longitudinal, and cross-over studies. The high and increasing consumption of sugars-sweetened drinks by children in many countries is of serious concern. It has been estimated that each additional can or glass of sugars-sweetened drink that they consume every day increases the risk of becoming obese by 60%.

Most of the evidence relates to soda drinks but many fruit drinks and cordials are equally energy-dense and may promote weight gain if drunk in large quantities. Overall, the evidence implicating a high intake of sugars-sweetened drinks in promoting weight gain was considered moderately strong.

Adverse socio-economic conditions, especially for women in high-income countries (causative): Classically the pattern of the progression of obesity through a population starts with middle-aged women in high-income groups but as the epidemic progresses, obesity becomes more common in people (especially women) in lower socio-economic status groups. The relationship may even be bi-directional, setting up a vicious cycle (i. e. lower socio-economic status promotes obesity, and obese people are more likely to end up in groups with low socio-economic status).

The mechanisms by which socio-economic status influences food and activity patterns are probably multiple and need elucidation. However, people living in circumstances of low socio-economic status may be more at the mercy of the obesogenic environment because their eating and activity behaviours are more likely to be the "default choices" on offer. The evidence for an effect of low socio-economic status on predisposing people to obesity is consistent (in higher income countries) across a number of cross-sectional and longitudinal studies, and was thus rated as a "probable" cause of increased risk of obesity.

Breast-feeding (protective): Breast-feeding as a protective factor against weight gain has been examined in at least 20 studies involving nearly 40,000 subjects. Five studies (including the two largest) found a protective effect, two found that breastfeeding predicted obesity, and the remainder found no relationships. There are probably multiple effects of confounding in these studies; however, the reduction in the risk of developing obesity observed in the two largest studies was substantial (20–37%). Promoting breastfeeding has many benefits, the prevention of childhood obesity probably being one of them.

Possible Etiological Factors

Several other factors were defined as "possible" protective or causative in the etiology of unhealthy weight gain. Low-glycaemic foods have been proposed as a potential protective factor against weight gain and there are some early studies that support this hypothesis. More clinical trials are, however, needed to establish the association with greater certainty. Large portion sizes are a possible causative factor for unhealthy weight gain. The marketing of "supersize" portions, particularly in fastfood outlets, is now common practice in many countries.

There is some evidence that people poorly estimate portion sizes and that subsequent energy compensation for a large meal is incomplete and therefore is likely to lead to over-consumption. In many countries, there has been a steady increase in the proportion of food eaten that is prepared outside the home. In the United States, the energy, total fat, saturated fat, cholesterol and sodium content of foods prepared outside the home is significantly higher than that of home-prepared food. People in the United States who tend to eat in restaurants have a higher BMI than those who tend to eat at home.

Certain psychological parameters of eating patterns may influence the risk of obesity. The "flexible restraint" pattern is associated with lower risk of weight gain, whereas the "rigid restraint/periodic disinhibition" pattern is associated with a higher risk. Several other factors were also considered but the evidence was not thought to be strong enough to warrant defining them as protective or causative. Studies have not shown consistent associations between alcohol intake and obesity despite the high energy density of the nutrient (7 kcal/g). There are probably many confounding factors that influence the association.

While a high eating frequency has been shown in some studies to have a negative relationship with energy intake and weight gain, the types of foods readily available as snack foods are often high in fat and a high consumption of foods of this type might predispose people to weight gain. The evidence regarding the impact of early nutrition on subsequent obesity is also mixed, with some studies showing relationships for high and low birth weights.

Strategies for Obesity Prevention

The prevention of obesity in infants and young children should be considered of high priority. For infants and young children, **the main preventive strategies are:**

a) The promotion of exclusive breastfeeding;

b) Avoiding the use of added sugars and starches when feeding formula;

c) Instructing mothers to accept their child's ability to regulate energy intake rather than feeding until the plate is empty;

d) Assuring the appropriate micronutrient intake needed to promote optimal linear growth.

For children and adolescents, prevention of obesity implies the need to:

a) Promote an active lifestyle;

b) Limit television viewing;

c) Promote the intake of fruits and vegetables;

d) Restrict the intake of energy-dense, micronutrient-poor-foods (e. g. packaged snacks);

e) Restrict the intake of sugars-sweetened soft drinks.

Additional measures include modifying the environment to enhance physical activity in schools and communities, creating more opportunities for family interaction (e. g. eating family meals), limiting the exposure of young children to heavy marketing practices of energydense, micronutrient-poor-foods, and providing the necessary information and skills to make healthy food choices. In developing countries, special attention should be given to avoidance of overfeeding stunted population groups.

Nutrition programmes designed to control or prevent undernutrition need to assess stature in combination with weight to prevent providing excess energy to children of low weight-for-age but normal weight-for-height. In countries in economic transition, as populations become more sedentary and able to access energy-dense foods, there is a need to maintain the healthy components of traditional diets (e. g. high intake of vegetables, fruits and NSP). Education provided to mothers and low socio-economic status communities that are food insecure should stress that overweight and obesity do not represent good health.

Low-income groups globally and populations in countries in economic transition often replace traditional micronutrient-rich-foods by heavily marketed, sugars-sweetened beverages (i. e. soft drinks) and energy dense fatty, salty and sugary foods. These trends, coupled with reduced physical activity, are associated with the rising prevalence of obesity. Strategies are needed to improve the quality of diets by increasing consumption of fruits and vegetables, in addition to increasing physical activity, in order to stem the epidemic of obesity and associated diseases.

Disease-specific Recommendations

Body Mass Index (BMI)

BMI can be used to estimate, albeit crudely, the prevalence of overweight and obesity within a population and the risks associated with it. It does not, however, account for the wide variations in obesity between different individuals and populations.

Waist Circumference

Waist circumference is a convenient and simple measure

which is unrelated to height, correlates closely with BMI and the ratio of waist-tohip circumference, and is an approximate index of intra-abdominal fat mass and total body fat. Furthermore, changes in waist circumference reflect changes in risk factors for cardiovascular disease and other forms of chronic diseases, even though the risks seem to vary in different populations. There is an increased risk of metabolic complications for men with a waist circumference $\geq 10^2$ cm, and women with a waist circumference ≥88 cm.

Physical Activity

A total of one hour per day of moderate-intensity activity, such as walking on most days of the week, is probably needed to maintain a healthy body weight, particularly for people with sedentary occupations.

Total Energy Intake

The fat and water content of foods are the main determinants of the energy density of the diet. A lower consumption of energy-dense (i. e. high-fat, high-sugars and high-starch) foods and energy-dense (i. e. high free sugars) drinks contributes to a reduction in total energy intake. Conversely, a higher intake of energy-dilute foods (i. e. vegetables and fruits) and foods high in NSP (i. e. wholegrain cereals) contributes to a reduction in total energy intake and an improvement in micronutrient intake. It should be noted, however, that very active groups who have diets high in vegetables, legumes, fruits and wholegrain cereals, may sustain a total fat intake of up to 35% without the risk of unhealthy weight gain.

9

FOOD AND DRUG ADMINISTRATION PLAN

Public health protection now includes addressing unprecedented challenges and threats to the health of the public-ones that are more sophisticated and complex than those of the last century. The FDA is dealing with new threats in the area of enforcement. Today, sophisticated criminals are increasingly targeting drugs, infant formula, and other FDA regulated products through well-organised operations. For example, recently the FDA has been investigating what appears to be a major operation selling a counterfeit version of a cholesterol-lowering drug. High-cost drugs present tempting targets for counterfeiters like those who put patients at risk by putting ordinary tap water into vials labeled as Procrit, a treatment for severe anemia.

The "drug" was contaminated with bacteria. Criminals are increasingly using the anonymity and reach of the Internet to get illegal drugs to potential customers. An investigation by the FDA's Office of Criminal Investigations led to the arrest of a man illegally distributing controlled substances through an Internet drug site-and this case represents just one of many similar cases of illegal Webbased pharmaceutical sales that the FDA has tackled and solved. In addition, rising health care costs have increased the stakes for frauds and kickbacks involving drugs and other medical products. An FDA investigation of sales and kickbacks related to a drug for prostate cancer helped uncover illegal activity that led to fines and payments of more than 350 million dollars.

The FDA's regulatory activities involve increasingly complex and rapidly changing production processes for medicines and foods. The FDA is also involved in preventing the spread of emerging infections, such as the recent outbreak of SARS, which are becoming more common as trade and travel have increased. At the same time, industry, government, and foundations are now spending unprecedented amounts of money to discover and develop new medical treatments $100 billion or more this year alone. And yet the number of new product applications submitted for FDA review has declined significantly, and in some cases precipitously.

In the pharmaceutical realm, last year the FDA filed 16 priority New Drug Applications (NDAs), down from a high of 32 in 1997. Standard NDA submissions are also down, as- 87 were filed last year, down from a high of 101 in 1999. Although the FDA is not responsible for the number and kinds of products in the development pipeline, the agency can foster and encourage new product development by ensuring that its review and approval processes are efficient, transparent, and predictable. We need to do more than ever to help make sure that the insights from biomedical science turn into safe and effective medical products more quickly, and at lower cost. The FDA has identified efficient risk management as the primary way to make the most effective use of agency resources and address these challenges.

Efficient risk management requires using the best scientific data, developing quality standards, and using efficient systems and practices that provide clear and consistent decisions and communications for the American public and regulated industry. The FDA has long led the way in the science of risk management, and this ability is more important than ever, given the expanding complexity of the agency's challenges and the need to reduce the health risks facing the public at the lowest possible cost to society. The principal objective of this strategic action plan is to do as much as possible to improve the health outcomes of the public. Only by becoming consistently more productive at what the agency does-always working to get the most public health bang for its regulatory buck-can the FDA have any chance of fulfilling its increasingly complex public health mission.

LIMITED RESOURCES FOR MAXIMUM PROTECTION

The number of medical products-drugs and devices, that the FDA regulates now exceeds 150,000 far more than ever before, including more complex products. There are almost 3,000 investigational new drugs under development, with their sponsors in the process of developing the evidence needed for FDA approval. There are more-and more diverse-dietary supplements on the market than ever before. Americans have a much broader range of food choices, including over 6 million food imports this year, with the import numbers growing rapidly. Access to this growing range of products offers opportunities for improving health and improving lives, but it also creates new kinds of vulnerabilities and risks to the public health.

Last year, the agency received some valuable new resources for carrying out its mission to enforce the laws to protect the food and drug supply. This included 800 additional personnel, most of them focused on assuring food safety and food security at border crossings, ports of entry, and analytical laboratories. With these resources, the agency has quintupled the number of food examinations it performs. Even with these additional resources, however, it is more important than ever for the FDA to use the best science and the best new enforcement ideas to carry out its increasingly challenging mission. The FDA's enforcement strategy consequently focuses on the most efficient way to get the most compliance with the law.

There are some key principles in the agency's science-based enforcement strategy:

- ***Clarity***: The FDA must develop and use clear and consistent guidance and communication with regulated firms to promote voluntary compliance with the law. Many businesses are willing to comply with science-based regulations, but in areas as complex as food and medical product manufacturing with technologies that are constantly changing, the FDA has found that assuring a company's understanding of regulatory requirements can substantially improve compliance.
- *Science*: The FDA must remain vigilant to ensure that its practices reflect and allow for the latest innovations in production, inspection, and enforcement techniques. The FDA's regulations should be no more burden some than necessary, and should encourage valuable innovation in foods and medical products.
- *Leverage*: As the FDA's mission has become broader and more complex, it is increasingly beneficial to work with partners, including other federal and state agencies as well as private oversight organisations, to bring more resources and a more coordinated, powerful approach to enforcement.
- ***Deterrence***: In conjunction with the use of clear,

science-based regulatory approaches, the FDA must also take effective action against those who deliberately engage in criminal activities or disregard the FDA's important regulations to promote public safety, including the use of punishments based on the most effective tools available, including enforcement actions and criminal prosecutions that will stand up in court.

DRUG DEVELOPMENT

By some estimates, it costs more than $800 million and typically takes well over a decade to develop a new drug; and by all estimates, the cost of developing safe and effective new medical products has increased greatly, more than doubling over the past decade. In addition, improvements in bio-medical science have not translated into a better success rate for investigational treatments. The vast majority of the treatments that enter clinical testing don't succeed. According to a recent analysis by researchers at Tufts, of all the new chemical entities that enter clinical testing, only 21.5 percent will achieve final clinical success and FDA marketing approval.

So may be it's not surprising that, on the one hand, there are more new medicines under investigation than ever before, but on the other hand, the number of truly new drugs (new molecular entities) approved by the FDA has been declining, down to 17 last year from a high of 53 in 1996 (figure 1). The decline in products approved isn't the result of the FDA rejecting more applications; it is directly related to the decline in the number of new applications coming in to the agency, and it is a worldwide phenomenon., There are a lot of reasons to think that this decline is temporary. It takes some time to turn all of the unprecedented public and private R&D investments now taking place into safe and effective treatments for patients.

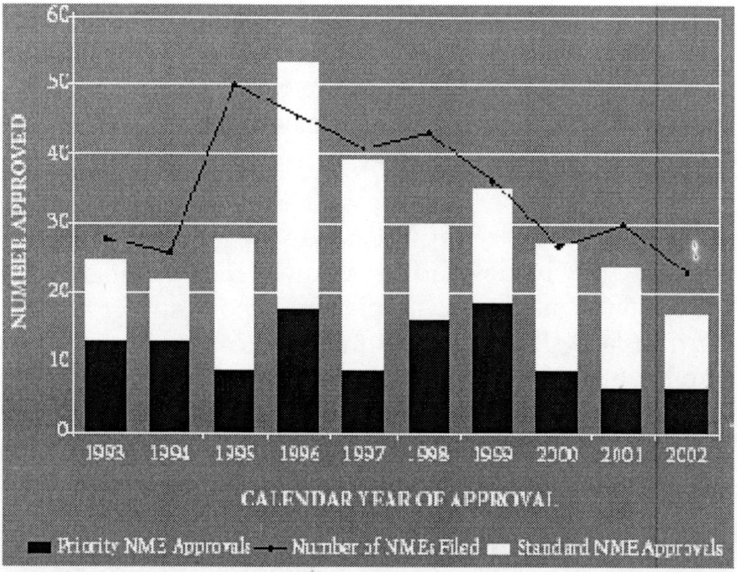

Figure 1: New Molecular Entity Approvals by Calendar Year

In particular, much of the growth in biomedical R&D has been devoted to new areas of product development, including genomics, proteomics, imaging and informational technologies, and many other areas. Because many of these new sciences are just beginning to emerge from laboratory and investigational settings, it seems plausible that the large new investments in biomedical R&D may take many years to pay off as an increase in the availability of safe and effective products for patients. This lengthy "translational" process means that it may still require some years and considerable additional costs before such an increase occurs.

However, rising costs of product development may be an important contributor to problems of rising health care costs and problems of timely access to the most effective modern treatments. Steps to reduce the time, cost, and uncertainty of developing new drugs and devices are thus important public health priorities. For example, the Tufts researchers estimate that drug companies can achieve a $200 million reduction in total development costs by reducing clinical phase times by 41 percent, or by increasing clinical success rates from the current 21.5 percent to approximately 31 percent.

Millions of peoples are suffering from diseases that may be curable or at least manageable as a result of technologies in development now. From a public health standpoint, making it simpler and more straightforward to translate all these investments into valuable products can have a substantial positive impact on the health of the nation, and can improve access to needed care as well. Making the process of translating new discoveries into safe and effective treatments more efficient and quick is thus a high priority for the FDA.

DRUG MANUFACTURING

Another application of the FDA's principle of efficient risk management is focused on the agency's current standards and guidance to industry on the way medical products are manufactured, known as "Current Good Manufacturing Practices." The CGMP regulations for drugs have not been updated in 25 years. Meanwhile, best practices in manufacturing technologies and methods have undergone significant progress over that time, particularly in other high-tech industries. For example, the semi-conductor industry also has a very low tolerance for impurities and inaccuracies in production.

Through continuous quality improvement, the semi-conductor industry achieved enormous improvements in production cost and quality, and these techniques have since been widely adopted in many manufacturing industries. But continuous quality improvement in manufacturing hasn't been the subject of as much attention in the pharmaceutical industry, even though many experts on manufacturing processes believe that large savings in production costs could be realised while maintaining very high standards for purity and accuracy.

The FDA wants to make sure that its regulations are encouraging such progress. So the FDA's broad-based programme is working on developing new guidance based on the latest science of risk management and quality assurance. The new standards are being designed to encourage cost-reducing and precision-enhancing innovation in manufacturing and technology, and to ensure that the FDA uses consistent and up-to-date methods, including inspectors specialising in particular types of production methods.

Chemical and Engineering News reports that, although pharmaceutical laboratories are working aggressively to produce new drugs, "Behind the scenes, the industry is hoping to boost its performance by cutting costs in areas it has basically ignored." Manufacturing had been on the bottom of the list of concerns for 15 years in pharmaceuticals and now it is a frontline issue.

Over the past decade, the number of FDA-regulated imports has increased dramatically. In the past 5 years alone, the number of import line entries has nearly doubled, growing from 4.2 million in 1997 to 7.8 million in 2002. Approximately two-thirds of these line entries are foods. Meanwhile, the FDA's capacity to examine imports physically has not kept pace with the significant growth in the number of imports of FDA-regulated products. The result is that by 2002, the FDA physically examined less than 1.3 percent of all entries offered for import into the United States. The FDA has compensated for the tremendous growth in its regulatory mission by working with international agencies that export FDA-regulated products to the United States to leverage off of their efforts, and by devoting significant new personnel resources to border examinations.

To further enhance import security with limited resources, the FDA is implementing new regulations to address threats, improve the agency's ability to target its field resources to imports that present the most significant risks, respond more quickly and effectively if an event involving an FDA-regulated product occurs, and collaborate with other government agencies and regulated firms to increase security and mitigate threats.

FOODBORNE DISEASE

The annual cost of foodborne illness is increasing year-by year. In USA, Officials of the Department of Health and Human Services project that the reported incidence of foodborne illness may increase by 10 to 15 percent during the next decade. And changes in production practices, centralised product distribution, environmental conditions, and food consumption patterns could be contributing to the emergence of new microbial threats to health. The Centers for Disease Control and Prevention (CDC) estimates that foodborne diseases cause about 76 million illnesses, 325,000 hospitalisations, and 5,000 deaths in the United States each year.

Even these figures may be low due to the number of foodborne illnesses that go unreported. Some experts estimate that over 40 million cases of foodborne illness go unreported each year. The FDA is committed to reducing the incidence of foodborne illness by greater use of efficient risk management techniques, such as hazard analysis and critical control point (HACCP) strategies. These efforts are an important part of the agency's strategic plan.

RISK MANAGEMENT

The agency's approach to efficient risk management

requires the use of the most current biomedical, managerial, and economic science, along with improved standards and FDA-industry communications. This strategy will reduce unnecessary regulatory burdens, improve compliance with the law, and achieve greater and faster improvements in public health through safer, more effective, and more affordable medical and food technologies. It includes more efficient development and review processes for a widening variety of drugs, medical devices, biologics, and food additives, while sustaining the FDA's gold standards for safety and effectiveness. It also includes using the best available data and analytic methods to assess risk and to develop the most effective approaches for inspections and other compliance and enforcement activities.

The FDA will be pursuing the most cost-effective allocation of its resources to identify food safety hazards and reduce illness and injury of food products. And the agency will work to make imports safer by using a risk-based system to inspections. The FDA's goal for efficient risk management includes **the following four objectives and strategies:**

a) Provide timely, high quality, cost-effective process for review of new technologies/ pre-market submissions. Reduce avoidable delays and costs in product approvals through clear expectations and effective communication of standards to sponsors by:

- Analysing root causes of multiple review cycles and establishing steps to prevent additional cycles when possible and
- Developing additional agency guidances on innovative and crosscutting product development where development pathways are particularly difficult or unclear.

Initiate the development of a continuous improvement/quality systems approach to the approval process throughout premarket review of new applications. Direct agency research programmes and develop standards to effectively handle emerging technologies, especially in areas of pharmacogenomics, gene therapy, and combination devices. The objective is more efficient and rapid translation of new scientific developments and break-throughs into safe and effective medical products.

b) Provide high quality, cost-effective oversight of industry manufacturing, processing and distribution to reduce risk. Apply the most current scientific knowledge about risk management and quality assurance to the FDA's requirements, including Current Good Manufacturing Practice (CGMP) inspection, compliance, and enforcement activities. Develop new inspection approaches to more effectively utilise new and existing resources. Implement an efficient, risk-based system to promote the wide availability of safe FDA-regulated imports by increasing the standards and improving the practices of source countries and at points of entry into U.S. commerce, improving detection of noncompliant products, and developing standards and procedures to maximise the cost-effectiveness of agency oversight.

c) Assure the safety of the U.S. food and cosmetics supply to protect consumers at the least cost for the public.

   – Develop and use new scientific knowledge and use public health systems to quickly and accurately identify food safety hazards so that disease risks can be properly managed. Identify appropriate prevention standards and apply appropriate preventive controls and inspection and monitoring systems to assure food safety for all Americans.

- Measure results regarding health outcomes to verify that foodborne illness and injury is being reduced.
- Consider risk information in deciding how to manage food imports, whether by: (1) working with foreign countries and manufacturers to improve compliance with safe manufacturing abroad as an alternative to detailed inspections at the border, (2) using better information on imports to focus border checks of final products that present significant potential risks, or (3) collaborating with domestic producers to improve checks on the safety of the ingredients they use.

d) Develop methodological strategies and analyses to evaluate options, identify the most effective and efficient risk management strategies, and optimise regulatory decision-making. Develop and evaluate strategies using scientific data to optimise premarket and postmarket regulatory decisions. Develop timely, first-rate integrated risk assessment and economic analysis to identify efficient risk management options for policy makers.

HEALTH THROUGH BETTER INFORMATION

For all that the FDA can accomplish through efforts to improve enforcement and regulatory protections for the public-as well as to help encourage the development of safer, more effective, and affordable food and medical technologies-people, through their own choices, can have an even greater impact on improving their health. As the prevalence of obesity continues to rise, the long-term health and economic consequences of obesity will be astounding.

Lack of physical activity and poor nutrition account for approximately 300,000 deaths each year, making these risk factors second only to tobacco use in causes of preventable death. It has been estimated that up to 48 percent of English-speaking patients in the United States lack functional health literacy-the ability of an individual to understand, access, and use health-related information and services. U.S. Surgeon General Richard H. Carmona recently recognised low health literacy as a widespread problem affecting public health preparedness, addressing health care disparities, and disease prevention.

Combined with the increasing incidence of many health problems, such as diabetes and obesity, this is a serious public health problem. Clearly, making sure that health information available to consumers is clear, informative, and effective in helping them to improve their health is more important than ever. And the importance of protecting consumers from misleading information is greater than ever as well.

From encouraging better guidance to patients in pharmacy labels, to giving clearer guidance on communicating risk and benefit information in direct-to-consumer advertising, to launching new enforcement initiatives against dietary supplement manufacturers who make health claims without scientific foundation, the FDA is undertaking major new efforts to help consumers make better-informed decisions about how to use their health care dollars.

Information that consumers and other stake-holders receive should be truthful and not misleading and should clearly indicate a product's benefits and risks and the limitations of the scientific certainty associated with its use. The FDA accomplishes this important task in a number of ways. First, the FDA takes steps to ensure that information provided by a product's sponsors is accurate and that it communicates information consumers need to know in order to safely use a product. Second, the FDA itself communicates directly with the public and through health care providers concerning risks and benefits of regulated products. The scope of this communications responsibility is especially significant when it comes to food, as the FDA regulates some 75 percent of all foods consumed here, and given the current national epidemic of obesity and the related consequences, such as heart disease and diabetes.

The FDA knows that consumers want the best information available about each of the products they use. And consumer research has demonstrated that more and better information helps consumers make smarter and better-informed decisions. A recent study by the Federal Trade Commission on peoples' interpretation of food nutrition and health claims in advertising found that people are able to accurately interpret these kinds of qualified claims, even in cases where there are limitations in scientific support, so long as the specific disclosures are clear and accurate.

Recent innovations, such as the new label on over-the-counter (OTC) drugs (Figure 2) and direct-to-consumer (DTC) advertising, have had positive effects on consumer health decision-making. For example, consumer research conducted in developing the OTC drug label showed that the new label would increase consumers' confidence in their ability to use the information on the label and better enable them to make correct product-use decisions. Yet the FDA also knows that information can at times be confusing to some consumers, and too much information can provide a cacophony of data that can obscure the most important facts. Obviously, scientific accuracy is a key element of effective communication for consumers.

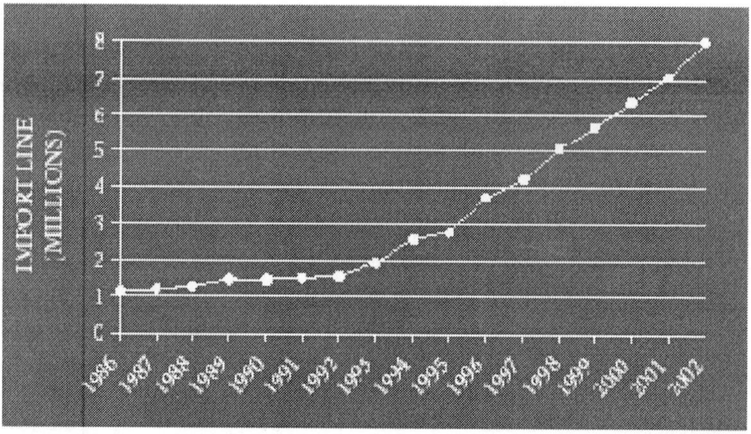

Figure 2. Growth of Imported Lines of Entry

Some other factors that affect the value of written medical information include, for example, the vocabulary and grammar used, the size of the typeface, and patient-related factors having to do with the patient's literacy. Consider the situation with the nutrition information on food products. Since 1993 consumers have been able to use the Nutrition Facts panel on food packages to help decide what foods to purchase. These labels were developed with the intent of enhancing the ability of peoples to make healthy diet choices. However, data on the health of Americans, particularly the growing problem of obesity, suggest that we are making dietary and other lifestyle choices that adversely affect our health despite access to this information.

The FDA's strategic plan calls for the agency to improve its knowledge about effective communications to consumers and health care providers throughout all of its major activities, including drugs, medical devices, and food products. The agency's current and future communication strategies for conveying risk, as well as the promotional activities of FDA sponsors, will be scientifically evaluated for their effectiveness in reaching target audiences and conveying information that is accurate and not misleading. The agency will be seeking out communications experts in academia, other government agencies, and industry to assist in these efforts. Other key strategies include:

Taking steps to improve the FDA's processes for reviewing industry communications to consumers and health care providers Enhancing the FDA's processes for reviewing message content and delivery Ensuring that critical health messages are being delivered in ways that meet the health needs of targeted groups, including the underserved and at-risk.

FDA's Objectives

Provide new important information on pediatric labeling to advocacy groups and health care providers. About 75 percent of all drugs prescribed for children are not tested for use in children, and as a result they may be ineffective or even harmful. The 2002 Best Pharmaceuticals for Children Act (BPCA) was intended to encourage the study of drug therapies in children. The BPCA also required public dissemination of important news about pediatric drug information and labeling changes.

Enhance the FDA's efforts to help ensure that industry communications to consumers and health care providers are truthful and not misleading, provide information about product risks and benefits, and appropriately convey the degree of scientific uncertainty associated with such product messages. A well-informed public is one of the best weapons against some of the biggest public health threats facing the country. Better information means that consumers can make better choices. And some of the most important health choices that people make are about the foods they choose to eat. Our choices about our diets are choices about our health.

Those choices should be based on the best and latest scientific information. One of the FDA's most important public health tasks is to help ensure that Americans can rely on that information to make smart decisions about food. To make these smart decisions, people need good, clear information about the nutritional value of their foods.

They also need to be protected from misleading information, from "snake oil" claims that create false hopes and can get in the way of improving their health. The Task Force on Consumer Health Information for Better Nutrition was charged, among other things, with developing a system for the FDA to help consumers get more accurate information about the health consequences of their food choices. The FDA believes that this process for making science-based health claims, when combined with the agency's strong enforcement work, will help people choose healthier products.

More effective enforcement of the law against companies that make false or misleading health claims also means that consumers can rely on the science-based information on the label. The health claims that the FDA believes are highest priority to go through this enhanced FDA-regulated process are the ones where the evidence seems quite good already-not definitively settled, but good enough that many expert organisations believe people should know about it in making their diet choices. The claims that the agency intends to review for possible inclusion on food labels in the months ahead include:

- Consuming 5 to 9 servings of fruits and vegetables a day may reduce your risk of cancer and other chronic illnesses
- Substituting foods that are high in unsaturated fats for foods high in saturated or trans fats (vegetable

oils instead of solid fats) may reduce your risk of heart disease

- A diet that features foods high in omega-3 fatty acids, or that substitutes tree nuts instead of proteins high in saturated fats, may reduce your risk of heart disease

In order to create an environment for good information, the agency is committed to aggressively pursuing those who make false and misleading claims. In 2002, the FDA inspected more than 80 dietary supplement firms, several of which voluntarily corrected identified violations. In February 2003, the FDA seized dietary supplements from a firm in Florida in light of illegal claims that the products would treat a variety of medical conditions, including prevention of cancer and treatment of arthritis.

More recently, the FDA worked with the FTC in May 2003 to crack down on Internet marketers of products claimed to protect against, treat, and even cure Severe Acute Respiratory Syndrome (SARS). Direct-to-Consumer (DTC) advertising has become an important source of patient information about prescription drugs. Research demonstrates that these ads can have a positive impact on patient/physician communications. For such advertising to best inform consumers, it must effectively communicate not just the potential benefits of the advertised prescription drug, but also potential risks, such as those associated with drug interactions and the specific health condition of the individual considering taking the drug.

Implement joint campaign with the CDC to educate the public and health care providers about antimicrobial resistance: Addressing the growing problem of resistance of antibiotics used to treat human illnesses, the FDA recently issued a final rule requiring that labeling for all systemic antibacterial drugs intended for human use include statements that the improper use of antibiotics will lead to drug-resistant bacterial strains. The rule encourages physicians to prescribe antibiotics only when clinically necessary, and to take the time to counsel their patients on the proper use of these drugs.

IMPROVING PATIENT AND CONSUMER SAFETY

All FDA-regulated products have risks and benefits, and the agency plays an important role in measuring and preventing the numerous injuries and deaths related to these products. Clearly, however, there is substantial room for improvement in preventing adverse events involving FDA-regulated products.

Too many peoples suffer from adverse events related to medical products, dietary supplements, and foods. Sometimes problems arise when medical products and dietary supplements are misused because consumers or doctors didn't have the right information about a new treatment. But adverse events that are preventable aren't just caused by human error.

Even with the best available data, products are sometimes found to have side effects that were not predictable or detectable in any clinical trials and other studies prior to product use in real-world conditions. Because virtually all medical therapies have side effects and risks, it is important for these side effects to be well understood so that the FDA can be sure that the benefits of the products we approve outweigh their risks. This includes improving the agency's ability to understand particular risks in specific populations, e.g., elderly patients and patients from particular demographic groups or carrying certain genes that may be associated with differences in risks.

More mortality, morbidity, and related costs could be avoided as the FDA improves the management of product-related risks. In the FDA's purview, there are more health- care-products than ever before and more people are using them. For example, it is estimated that our pharmacists will fill 3.1 billion prescriptions by the end of this year; that's 60 percent more than 10 years ago. Detection of adverse events that cause harm and human suffering needs to be improved.

The FDA has always relied on "spontaneous" reporting systems to monitor the safety of a new medical product. Avoiding serious adverse events often means the FDA is dependent on astute doctors identifying problems with new drugs early enough to do something about it, whether that means warning doctors and patients to be extra vigilant for a potential problem, or in some cases, withdrawing drugs too dangerous to be safely used.

While these systems are effective in identifying rare and often serious adverse events, their reliance on health care providers and incomplete reporting means that appropriate detection and response to adverse events may be less timely and effective than is desirable. The agency needs to improve its systems for reporting safety problems. One way is to improve the quality and standardisation of the adverse event reports that the agency receives through the FDA's spontaneous adverse event reporting systems, and the agency is taking steps to do that.

Another very promising new way is to have direct and secure access to relevant electronic health information. Increasingly, health care providers are using computerised systems to store patient information, such as electronic medical records. Some of the information entered in these systems is related to product use and product-related adverse events.

Confidential, secure exchange of relevant information with these health care pro-vider systems could help to automate the discovery and reporting of safety problems. However, the use of different technology platforms and applications hampers the flow of information among these systems. The agency will work with its partners to develop standards to improve the flow of information across systems. In turn, it will increase the payoff to health care organisations from adopting electronic medical record systems, in the form of higher-quality and more timely electronic information from the FDA on product risks and benefits.

The agency will identify the most innovative and effective ways to better communicate the risks associated with regulated products. There is also an increasing number of health care databases available to study the use and outcomes associated with medical products. The agency has the challenge and the opportunity to use the best available information from the private and public sector to improve its understanding of product safety.

IMPROVING CONSUMER AND PATIENT SAFETY

FDA's Objectives are the following:

a) Enhance the ability to quickly identify risks associated with FDA-regulated products. The FDA will supplement the current passive reporting system by developing new ways to identify safety problems with medical products, dietary supplements and foods. This will speed up the process of recognising safety problems and allow for prevention of similar adverse events. Partnerships with health care providers and the CDC will allow the FDA to link to medical records and other public health monitoring systems to identify adverse events quickly. This means, for instance, if a drug were causing problems in a few patients' kidneys it would be detected early and managed before other patients risk injury.

b) Increase capacity to accurately analyse risks associated with medical products, dietary supplements, and foods. There are many different sources of information that the FDA will seek from other agencies and health care organisations to get a better understanding of how common an avoidable adverse event is and the severity of the problems associated with the product. The latest advances in statistics will also help analysts assess safety problems with FDA-regulated products. New computer software and specialised training will provide staff with the tools they need. These efforts will give the FDA the information needed to effectively protect public health.

c) Take appropriate actions to communicate risks and correct problems associated with medical products, dietary supplements and foods. The FDA will identify new ways to inform physicians, pharmacists, nurses, and patients about the safety of FDA-regulated products.

EFFECTIVE REGULATION THROUGH A WORKFORCE

One aspect of the FDA's work has remained, and will remain, unchanged: the critical importance of the FDA's professional workforce for the success of the agency and for its ability to maintain the high level of public trust in its activities. An organisation that can keep up with the rapid changes in the industries that it regulates, and is capable of developing and implementing effective and innovative public health measures, requires a very special workforce. The agency's mission depends more than ever on a solid cadre of experienced physicians, toxicologists, chemists, statisticians, mathematicians and other highly qualified and dedicated professionals. Their expertise is essential for making the FDA's regulatory decisions balanced and fair, and for keeping the agency on the cutting edge of the technology and sciences used in medicines, foods, and the other products the FDA regulates.

As the FDA's regulatory mission grows more complex, it is only by becoming consistently more efficient, seeking opportunities to improve its own management, and realising the efficiencies to be gained from improvements in organisation, infrastructure, and information technology, that the agency can continue to accomplish its growing and diverse mission with excellence. The FDA's principal tool for achieving all of these goals is its workforce. Unlike most other public health agencies, the FDA does not achieve its health mission through grants or financing health-related services. Instead, the FDA's principal public health resource is its professional staff. There are almost 1,500 people with Ph.D.'s at the FDA and more than 400 with medical degrees.

The money that the FDA is appropriated each year for its mission primarily gets spent at the FDA on this staff. Two-thirds of the FDA's budget is spent on its workforce. The FDA's contributions are primarily a reflection of its professional services. Some objectives of FDA's are following,

Ensure a high quality, diverse and motivated workforce: To attract and keep high-caliber employees who are responsive to the changing needs of the agency, the FDA needs to be responsive to their diverse needs. There are some reasons to be concerned about whether the FDA is doing enough to attract and develop the workforce it needs. For example, a recent GAO analysis found that the FDA's attrition rates for many of the people involved in its drug review process are higher than those for other federal public health agencies and the federal government as a whole.

The FDA has already undertaken many innovative and successful initiatives to address its workforce goals. The agency's employees can take advantage of flexible work schedules, including an "any-80" programme that can fit the difficult schedules of two working parents, care for sick kids and elderly parents, and other outside commitments. About one-fifth of FDA employees take advantage of the agency's flexi-placing programme, which permits telecommuting. The FDA supports employees with childcare, elder care, and other distinctive needs. In a recent survey conducted by OPM to gauge how federal employees feel about their jobs, the FDA did very well compared to other government agencies and the private sector, especially in how its employees feel that their individual work here relates to the agency's core mission.

About 73 percent said that they found the FDA a friendly place to work, 82 percent said their supervisor supports their need to balance work and family issues, and 65 percent said they would recommend the FDA as a place to work. The agency is doing well, and it wants to do better. But FDA employees develop skills that are in great demand in the private sector. In addition, more than 30 percent of the agency's workforce will be eligible for retirement in less than five years. So the FDA is working to develop succession plans and career development plans. The agency is expanding career options, such as new fellowships and part-time appointments at its devices center, to support combining work at the FDA with work in an academic job.

Specifically, the FDA is committed to creating a working environment and culture in which its product review officers have the opportunity for professional training, and in which review responsibilities are balanced with professional development. To foster the development of a new generation of leaders, the agency will increase its participation in existing formal and informal training programmes such as the HHS Emerging Leaders programme and FDA internship and mentoring programmes. The agency will also develop better programmes for career progression and identify targeted career tracks tailored for reviewers, compliance officers, investigators and administrative staff.

Increase efficiency and effectiveness of agency management: To maintain and strengthen its position as a premier public health agency, the FDA will modernise and update many of its administrative support services and ensure the accountability of its administrative support programmes to support the needs of agency staff. To accomplish these goals, the agency will adopt new management practices, such as: consolidating the delivery of administrative services using internal performance contracts, reviewing commercial jobs inside the agency (Full Time Equivalents or FTEs) to find those amenable for outsourcing improving information technology capabilities to boost productivity enhancing the agency's financial management to provide tighter control of revenues and expenditures integrating performance and budget information to support smarter resource decisions. The FDA intends to implement all of these changes with careful attention to the needs of the agency's staff and plans to implement methods for measuring how it is performing in achieving these goals.

Ensure effective communication and working relationships with key external stakeholders to enhance U.S. and global health outcomes: The FDA is working hard to reduce risks to public health from diseases, and from the products to help people avoid diseases and their complications. But the FDA cannot ensure that the public gets the maximum health benefits with minimum risks by working alone. The agency relies upon a national and global network of health, regulatory, and science partners, as well as industry representatives and other stakeholders. The FDA is committed to providing accurate, science-based information on the risks and benefits of the products it regulates to all those who use them, and to gathering information from all those who will help the agency ensure that FDA regulated products are safely used.

The FDA must communicate information about these risks in an accurate and timely manner. And the agency must have productive relationships with its partners to plan, implement and evaluate its risk management strategies. In addition, effective communication about FDA regulatory and enforcement policies can help make sure that regulated firms are doing all they can to protect and advance the health of the public. By working closely with partners in risk management, the FDA's ability to closely manage the risk associated with the products the FDA regulates is greatly improved. The FDA's stakeholder communities are many and varied, and collaborating with all of them creates the best opportunities for ensuring good health outcomes.

Transition Information technology from an enabler to a strategic tool for realising the FDA's policy goals and objectives: Currently, the FDA views Information Technology (IT) resources as a means for the agency's medical review staff to accomplish their day-to-day work. Information technologies help staff manage the volumes of information that the agency receives more efficiently, by minimising storage and administrative overhead, for example.

In the future, the FDA is going to view IT as a strategic tool that can be used by programme staff to accomplish their policy goals and objectives with greater efficiency and effectiveness. One key action item for the FDA is the development of an integrated IT process for determining and managing Center-unique systems, FDA-wide systems, and HHS-wide systems.

The FDA's blueprint calls for an IT capability that contributes directly to mission-critical goals, such as faster review of new drugs and medical devices, more rapid targeting of suspect imports, and quicker identification, analysis, and communication of medical errors and suspected problems with the use of new medical technologies.

Provide a consolidated FDA headquarters campus to improve operations for employees: The FDA is cooperating with the General Services Administration (GSA) to consolidate the agency's diverse headquarters components, now housed in over 40 different buildings all around the greater Washington, D.C., area, to a new campus at White Oak in Montgomery County, Md. This consolidation was initiated through the FDA Revitalisation Act of 1990, and the FDA is now making it reality. The new White Oak campus will begin housing employees in the coming year, and will house 1,700 FDA staff by 2005. There are four additional projects moving forward simultaneously at the White Oak campus, which together will eventually house a total of over 7,000 FDA employees in modern office and lab space.

The first FDA employees will be arriving at White Oak this fall. The consolidation of FDA headquarters from 16 locations to three will offer many benefits:

- Support effective collaboration and coordination of the agency's growing and diverse expertise in the face of increasingly complex public health challenges.
- Provide greater access to the public, as well as better security for agency personnel.

- Improve the efficiency of agency operations substantially through:
  - a) Standardised, modernised, and centralised document handling,
  - b) Greater use of shared facilities such as libraries and conference areas, and
  - c) Elimination of redundancies in a wide range of administrative management tasks
- Reduce management layers.
- Provide more of a "critical mass" for the agency's ability to develop and conduct scientific activities, including analyses for efficient risk management and translational and regulatory research, to improve the scientific foundations and efficiency of the FDA's regulatory activities.

10

POVERTY AND OBESITY

The content of school lunches has been scrutinised, and even food-assistance programmes have come under attack for their alleged role in "fattening the poor". Public-health-policies for the prevention of obesity increasingly call for taxes and levies on fats and sweets, both to discourage their consumption and to help promote alternative and healthier food choices.

POVERTY AND OBESITY

Among women, higher obesity rates tend to be associated with low incomes and low education levels. The association of obesity with low Socio-Economic Status (SES) has been less consistent among men. Minority populations (except for Asian Americans) have higher rates of obesity and overweight than do US whites. The relation between obesity and education and income, based on charts published by the Centers for Disease Control and Prevention.

Food insecurity and obesity also appear to be linked. The concept of food insecurity, originally adapted from work by the Food and Agriculture Organisation of the United Nations, was used to examine access to food by low-income households.

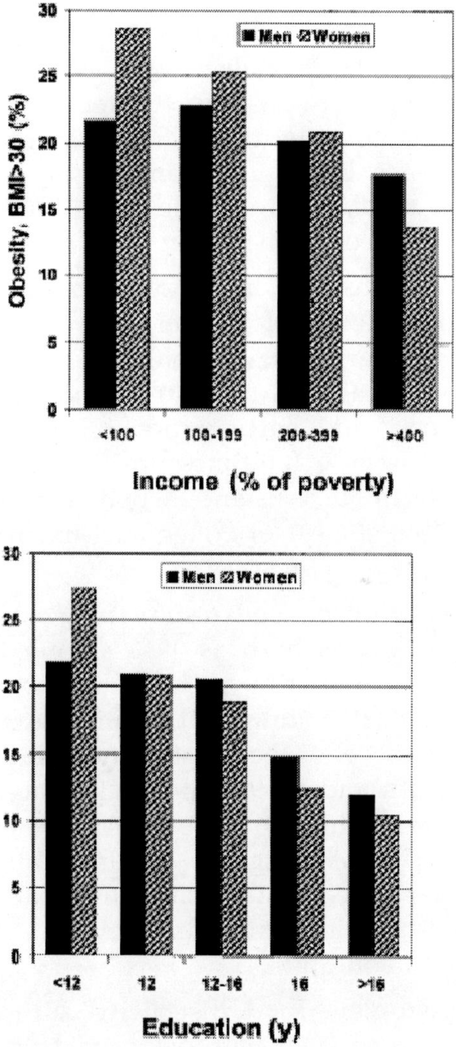

Figure 1: Obesity as a function of income and education.

In the 1995 US Department of Agriculture (USDA) Current Population Survey, food insecurity was defined as "limited or uncertain availability of nutritionally acceptable or safe foods". The 1995 Current Population Survey judged 11.9% of all US households to be food insecure. However, not all food-insecure households showed evidence of hunger, and the relation between poverty, food insecurity, and hunger was a complex one. There was no one-to-one correspondence between income-based measures of poverty and food insecurity, and only 13.1% of those in poverty were affected by hunger.

Of the food-insecure households, 65% (7.8% of total) showed no evidence of hunger, 28% (3.3%) reported moderate hunger, and 6.9% (0.8%) reported severe hunger. There was also a positive association between food insecurity and participation in the Food Stamp Programme, because food-insecure persons were more likely to seek food assistance. Food insufficiency was defined as "sometimes" or "often" not having enough to eat.

The prevalence of food insufficiency was 4% in the total sample but as high as 14% among low-income respondents. According to the USDA Economic Research Service, 10.1% (10.5 million) of American households reported some level of food insecurity in 1999, including 9.5% of adults and 16.9% of children aged < 18 y. Households with children were twice as likely to report food insecurity. Among low-income families, food insufficiency was associated with single-parent families, not having health insurance, and having a family head with < 12 y of education.

Among women, food insecurity without hunger appears to be associated with overweight. Food-insecure women were >10lb heavier on average than was the comparison group. Whereas links between food insecurity and lower diet quality might be expected, the association between food insecurity and overweight was something of a paradox.

ENERGY-DENSITY

In 1992, Basiotis hypothesised and confirmed a behavioural model in which household members faced with diminishing incomes first consumed less expensive foods to maintain energy intakes at a lower cost.

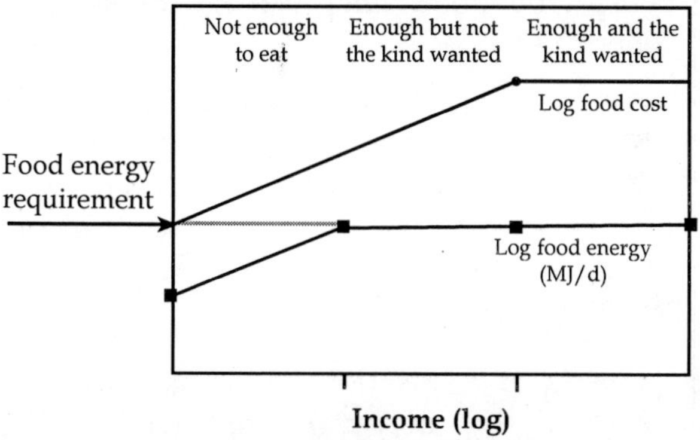

Figure 2: Food-insufficiency

To multiple-choice questions about food sufficiency, these participants responded "enough but not the kinds of food we want to eat", which implied adequate energy intakes but a limited range of food choices. Only when incomes diminished still further did households reduce dietary energy to intakes below daily requirements, which resulted in overt deprivation.

The food-insufficiency curve, linking household incomes with food costs and energy intakes, is shown in Figure 2. Food restriction at home first occurs in adults because parents typically turn over their own food to children when resources are scarce. The association between poverty and obesity is mediated, at least in part, by the low cost of energy-dense foods, which may in turn promote over-consumption.

The hypothesis is that energy density (MJ/kg) and

energy costs ($/MJ) are inversely linked, such that the selection of energy-dense foods by food-insecure or low-income consumers may represent a deliberate strategy to save money. Analogous to the findings of Basiotis, persons attempting to limit food costs will first select less expensive but more energy dense foods to maintain dietary energy.

The energy-cost curve linking food costs with dietary energy density and energy intakes is shown in Figure 3. As food costs diminish further, dietary energy density rises, and total energy intakes may actually increase.

INFLUENCES OF ENERGY DENSITY

Energy density of foods (MJ/kg) is said to be the key influence on daily energy intakes. Under laboratory conditions, people consume a constant volume of food at a given meal such that the energy density of foods determines the amount of energy consumed.

Palatable energy-dense foods have been associated with diminished satiation and satiety, "passive over-consumption" of fats and sweets, and higher energy intakes overall. In contrast, bulky foods with a high water content are said to promote a feeling of fullness, which leads to reduced energy intakes both at the test meal and throughout the day.

The energy density of foods is a function of their water content. Whereas energy-dilute foods are heavily hydrated, energy-dense foods are dry and may also contain fat, sugar, or starch. Potato chips (23 kJ/g), chocolate, and doughnuts (18 kJ/g) are energy-dense foods. Dairy products vary in energy density, from dry cheeses (17.0 kJ/g) to yogurt (4.2 kJ/g) to fluid low-fat milk (1.6 kJ/g).

Because of their high water content, the energy

density of raw vegetables and fruit is low (≈0.4 - 2.0 kJ/g). Beverages with different nutrient compositions may have the same energy density; for example, the energy density of 1% milk, orange juice, and cola is 1.8 kJ/g. Water contained in foods has a more pronounced effect on satiety than does water contained in beverages. Foods with a high moisture content, such as vegetables and fruit, allow the consumer to "feel full on fewer calories".

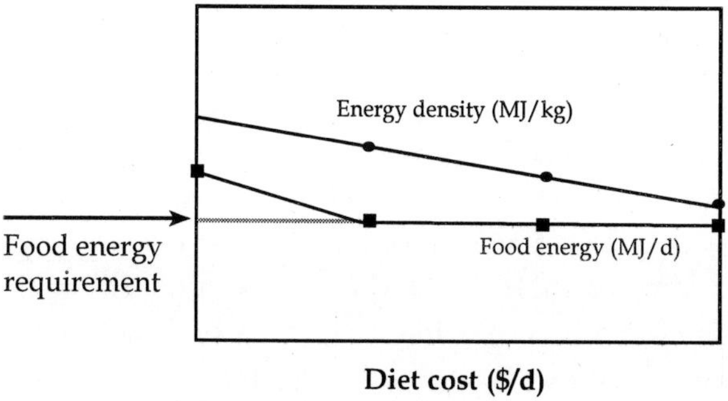

Figure 3: Energy density-cost

Whereas the energy density of foods can be obtained from nutrient-composition tables, calculation of the energy density of the total diet is more difficult. Such calculations generally include all foods and caloric beverages but exclude noncaloric beverages and water. In some cases, both caloric and noncaloric beverages were excluded. High-energy density diets are those that include more fast foods, snacks, and desserts, whereas diets lower in energy density are those that are higher in vegetables and fruit.

Higher dietary energy density tends to be positively associated with total energy intakes and with the percentage of energy from fat. The energy density of the children's diets was inversely associated with the percentage of energy from sugars, most likely because of the high consumption of energy-dilute soft drinks.

However, the relation between dietary energy density and overweight has been difficult to establish, given that it is confounded by age and energy expenditure.

High energy intakes in cross-sectional studies need not be evidence of hyperphagia, but may reflect the higher energy intakes of younger or more active persons. No community-based data have shown a causal connection between dietary energy density and overweight.

ENERGY-DENSE FOODS

Energy-dense foods are more palatable. Studies using laboratory animals have found sugar and fat to be powerful sources of neurobiological reward. Foods that are energy-dense provide more sensory enjoyment and more pleasure than do foods that are not. Clinical studies suggest that the most likely targets of food cravings are those foods that contain fat, sugar, or both. In times of dietary scarcity, human preferences for energy-dense foods represented an advantage in survival.

Human taste preferences for sugar and fat are either innate or acquired very early in life. Studies with children have consistently shown that familiarity, sweetness, and energy density are the chief determinants of food preference. Very young children learn to prefer novel nonsweet flavours once the flavours have been associated with a concentrated source of energy, such as starch or fat.

Studies of the food preferences of 3-4-y-old children showed that preferences were driven by familiarity and the energy density of the foods. Children preferred the more energy-dense foods and gave higher ratings to chocolate cookies and potato chips than to vegetables and fruits. Preferences can also be shaped by repeated exposures or by a positive association with postingestive metabolic consequences of a food. Mothers may also influence children's food choices through their own preferences.

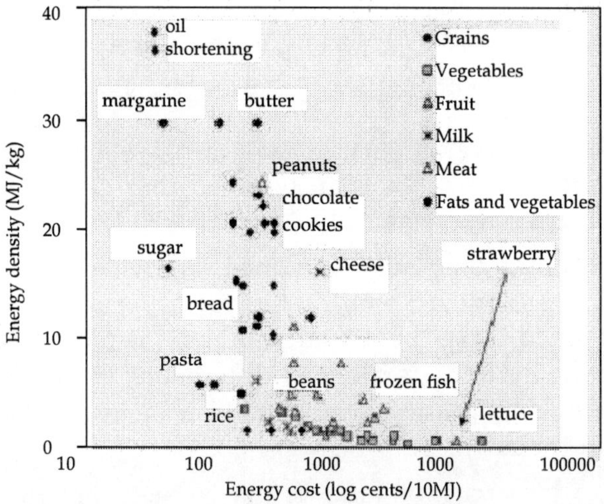

Figure 4: Relation between the energy density of selected foods and energy costs

Mothers indicated that their children liked energy-dense foods such as pizza, chocolate, chips cookies, and sweetened breakfast cereals, whereas low-energy-density tomatoes, cucumbers, and cabbage were disliked by children and their mothers. Whether induced by innate taste preferences, early exposure, or other environmental factors, long-term dietary exposure to sugar and fat may have permanent metabolic consequences on the organism.

Low Energy Costs

High energy density means low energy costs. Developments in agriculture and food technology have made energy-dense foods accessible to consumers at a very low cost. The relation between the energy density of selected foods and their energy cost is shown in Figure 4.

Energy density values were taken from food composition tables and from Rolls and Barnett, whereas energy costs were based on super-market prices in Seattle collected in the winter of 2003. According to the figure, energy cost of cookies or potato chips was ≈20 cents/MJ (1200 kcal/$), whereas that of fresh carrots was ≈95 cents/MJ (250-kcal/$). The energy cost of soft drinks was, on average, 30- cents/MJ (875 kcal/$), whereas that of orange juice from concentrate was 143 cents/MJ (170 kcal/$).

Fats and oils, sugar, refined grains, potatoes, and beans represented some of the lowest-cost options and provided dietary energy at minimal cost. As indicated by the logarithmic scale, the differential in energy costs between sugar and strawberries was in the order of several thousand percent.

The hierarchy of food prices is such that dry foods with a stable shelf life are generally less costly (per MJ) than are perishable meats or fresh produce with a high water content. As a rule, potato chips, chocolate, and locally bottled soft drinks provide dietary energy at a lower cost than do naturally hydrated lean meats, fish, and fresh vegetables and fruit. Energy-dense foods may contain a relatively high proportion of refined grains, added sugars, and vegetable fats.

The current US diet derives close to 50% of energy from added sugars and fat. Data from the Economic Research Service of the USDA show that the per capita availability of caloric sweeteners and fats and oils each increased by ≈20% between 1977 and 1997. Retail price increases during that time were much lower for sweets and fats than for vegetables and fruits.

Other studies have shown that foods identified as accounting for the greatest increase in energy intake by Americans during that time were salty snacks, desserts, soft drinks, fruit drinks, hamburgers and cheese-burgers,

Mexican food, and pizza. In 1977-1978, these foods combined accounted for 18.1% of the dietary energy consumed by Americans (> 2y) and for 27.7% of energy in 1994-1996. For the most part, many such foods are composed of refined grains, added sugars, and fats.

Studies on dietary choices leading to obesity have focused overwhelmingly on the sugar and fat content of snacks, fast foods, beverages, and confectionery. Epidemiologic studies have linked diets composed of fats and sweets, potatoes, and refined grains with higher glycemic indexes and a higher risk of obesity and type 2 diabetes.

Obese patients were accordingly advised to replace fats and sweets with a more prudent dietary pattern characterised by a high intake of fruits, vegetables, whole grains, poultry, and fish. Among public health measures for the prevention of obesity are the need to restrict the consumption of energy-dense snacks and sugar-sweetened soft drinks and to increase the consumption of whole grains and energy-dilute vegetables and fruit.

The inverse relation between energy-density and energy cost suggests that "obesity-promoting" foods are simply those that offer the most dietary energy at the lowest cost. Given the differential in energy costs between energy-dense and energy-dilute foods, the advice to replace fats and sweets with fresh vegetables and fruit may have unintended economic consequences for the consumer.

Prices and incomes affect food choices, dietary habits, and diet quality. The Healthy Eating Index (HEI)-a 10-component, 100-points scale developed by the USDA-is a measure of the quality of the total diet. The first 5 components measure the degree to which a given diet conforms to the food guide pyramid in the consumption of grains, vegetables, fruits, milk products, and meat. The next 5 components measure fat, saturated fat, cholesterol, and sodium intakes as well as the variety of foods in the diet. An HEI score of 80 implies a "good" diet, a score between 51 and 80 implies that a diet "needs improvement," and a score < 51 indicates a "poor" diet.

Income disparities had more of an effect on diet quality than on total energy intakes. HEI scores were typically higher for women than for men and improved with increasing age, education, and income. Education had a stronger effect on diet quality than did incomes. Although African Americans had the lowest HEI scores, scores for Latinos and Asians were no different from those for whites.

Strong associations between higher household incomes and higher quality diets were also obtained in studies conducted in Canada, France, the United Kingdom, and other countries of the European Union. Women reporting food insufficiency had lower quality diets. Mean HEI scores in the 1988-1994 NHANES III data set were 58.8 for women in food-insufficient households compared with 62.7 for women in food-sufficient households.

Food-insufficient women had lower HEI component scores for fruit (2.2 compared with 3.4), vegetables (5.1 compared with 5.8), milk (5.2 compared with 6.1), and food variety (6.4. compared with 7.3) and were less likely to comply with the cholesterol guidelines (7.4 compared with 8.2). Women in food-insufficient households consumed the same amount of energy as did women in food-sufficient households.

Although the energy density of the diet was not calculated, energy-dense diets are those that contain the least fruit, vegetables, and milk. Limited economic resources appeared to have an adverse effect, not so much on dietary energy, but rather on the overall quality and, potentially, the energy density of the diet.

Health disparities among US population groups are related to inequalities in SES. Some of these disparities may be mediated by an unequal access to a healthy diet. Whereas "good" diets were associated with higher education and incomes, "poor" diets were associated with overweight. In USDA studies, female CSFII respondents aged > 19y with "poor" diets had a BMI of 26.4 compared with 24.8 for females whose diets were "good". For males, "poor" diets were associated with a BMI of 26.8, as opposed to 25.7 for "good" diets.

The effect of SES variables on diet quality has normally been ascribed to a higher educational level or to a greater awareness of health issues among higher-income respondents. However, nutrition knowledge alone does not necessarily lead to a healthy diet. Another possibility is that healthier diets cost more and are beyond the reach of many low-income families.

Data from the Bureau of Labour Statistics indicate that income disparities do affect diet quality. Food purchases made by high-income households differed markedly from those made by low-income households. In 1992, households in the top quintile by income spent Rs. 89865/ person (2.6% of total expenditures) for food, compared with Rs. 56205 (18.7%) spent by those in the bottom quintile.

Wealthier households bought higher-quality meats, more fish and seafood, more fruits and vegetables, and more convenience foods. Despite buying lower-cost items, poor households devoted a far greater share of their disposable income to food. Their level of satisfaction with the perceived quality of the diet was not reported. To achieve a healthy diet it may be necessary to spend more money. The UK Women's Cohort Study is one of the few observational studies to have explored food costs, perceived and actual, in a study cohort of 15, 191 women aged 35-69 y.

Women in the healthiest diet group spent an additional 617 pounds sterling per year on food relative to the least-healthy diet group, with vegetables and fruits accounting for the largest amount of the cost. Yet almost 71% in the healthiest diet group and 60% in the least-healthy group did not agree that it was more expensive to eat a healthier diet, contrary to evidence obtained from the study itself. The individual assessment of diet costs was, to a large extent, a matter of subjective perception rather than of objective facts.

There is substantial evidence that food purchases are influenced by food costs. Several studies have mentioned diet costs as a barrier to dietary change, especially among low-income respondents. Dietary variety and the consumption of fresh produce were generally associated with higher food costs. In USDA studies, total energy intakes or percentage of energy from fat varied little with incomes or participation in the Food Stamp Programme (FSP).

In contrast, a greater dietary variety and higher consumption of vegetables and fruit were associated with higher education and higher income levels. Recent USDA/ Economic Research Service analyses of food and nutrient intakes by income, defined in relation to poverty status, showed the same link between incomes and diet quality. Although there was not much difference in energy or macronutrient intakes by income and no difference in the consumption of basic commodities (milk, meat, and grains), there were major incomerelated differences in the consumption of (among other foods) lettuce and lettuce-based salads; melons, berries, and other fruits; and carbonated sodas.

The proportion of women consuming salads and

fruits on a given day was double for the highest-income group (>350% poverty) relative to the lower-income group (<131% poverty). Observational data on the costs of freely chosen diets are limited. The USDA CSFII provides data on individual food consumption and nutrient intakes. The Consumer Expenditure Survey does not report quantities of foods purchased, whereas the CSFII does not collect data on the cost of the foods consumed. Neither database can provide information about diet quality in relation to diet costs.

The USDA Food Stamp Survey does report food use and food price data but it is limited to food-assistance recipients. Further studies on diet quality in relation to diet costs represent a major research need. As yet, there are no data that would allow us to link all of the dietary and economic variables into a causal chain. In the absence of large-scale community studies, few intervention studies purport to show that healthful diets are not more expensive than are less healthful diets.

One study, based on only 20 families with an obese 8-12-y-old child undergoing treatment, and a high attrition rate showed that a decrease in family energy intakes from 1881 to 1338 kcal/person was indeed associated with a decrease in diet costs from Rs.305 to Rs.227. However, energy costs per 1000 kcal actually increased by > 10%. Nonetheless, the authors concluded that a more healthful diet was not more expensive than the typical American diet.

The share of income spent on food decreases as incomes increase. Because incomes have increased faster than food costs, average food expenditures in the United States have dropped to only 10.7% of incomes in 1997. In 1997, Americans spent 9.4% of their disposable income on foods consumed at home but only 6.6% in 1997. Percentage expenditures on foods away from home decreased slightly from 4.2% to 4.1%. The drop in food spending was disproportionately greater than the drop in spending on other goods.

By 1999, total daily expenditures on foods and beverages (including alcohol) were estimated at just under Rs. 360 per person. Assuming a daily ration of 10.5 MJ (2500 kcal), the estimated mean energy cost of the total diet was 76.9 cents/MJ. Other USDA estimates of the mean energy costs of the American diet were even lower, at 41.6 cents/MJ. Among industrialised nations, lower energy costs are generally associated with higher energy intakes.

The corollary of Engel's Law is that low-income families spend a higher proportion of disposable income on food. Whereas households with incomes> Rs. 3,150,000/y spent 7% of after-taxes income on food, low-income families spent close to 25%. Food costs were an issue, especially for low-income families and elderly female respondents. Focus groups conducted with FSP participants reported that all groups reported food price as the most important consideration in making food choices. The most important factor in choosing and preparing foods was to ensure that no one would complain they are still hungry.

Economic factors may help explain why low-income respondents are least likely to eat healthy diets and suffer from some of the highest rates of obesity and type 2 diabetes. Consuming energy-dense foods, and energy-dense diets, is an important strategy used by low-income consumers to stretch the food budget. Energy-dense foods carry a lower price tag, which allows for a higher energy consumption at a lower cost. Energy-dense foods also tend to be well-liked, even perceived as a reward, a factor that would reinforce their initial selection and repeated consumption. In general, taste is rated ahead of health and variety as an influence on food purchases and consumption patterns.

Diet composition after the imposition of cost constraints. One obstacle is posed by the lack of large data sets on food prices or food expenditures. In the absence of food-expenditures data, the USDA used mean national food prices based on the 1989 CSFII to estimate diet costs. That calculation served as the basis for the USDA Thrifty Food Plan (TFP), a national standard for a nutritious diet at a minimal cost that is used as the basis for food stamp allotments.

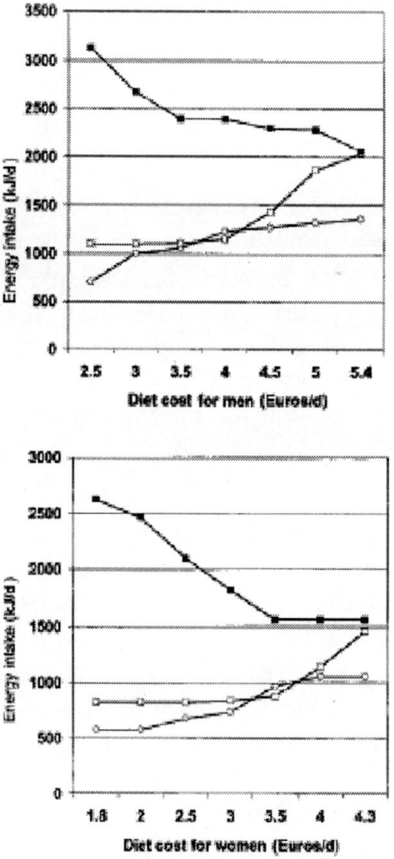

Figure 5: Change in energy intakes from different food sources in men and women.

The TFP "market basket" is composed of 44 foods, is based on a mathematical optimisation model that uses as inputs food guide pyramid servings, average daily consumption, nutrient composition of foods, and the average food price. Each TFP market basket identified the type and quantity of foods that people in different groups, by sex and age, might consume to achieve a healthful diet.

The foods were selected by using a nonlinear programming model that selected diets meeting specified nutritional criteria, with individual foods subject to cost constraints. Palatability was considered, but foods were not optimised for this objective. Given nutritional and cost constraints, the recommended foods featured grains and legumes, low-cost meats, and added sugars and fat.

Among the foods recommended for a week for a family of 4 were potatoes, pasta and rice (6 lb, 2722 g), beans (3 lb, 1361 g), bread (3 lb, 1361 g), sugar (1 lb, 454 g), lemonade (1 gallon, 3.8 L), added fats (2 lb, 907g), frozen turkey (5 lb, 2268 g), and frozen orange juice (6 lb, 2722 g). The allotment of leaf lettuce was 4 oz (113 g)/wk, which reflects sharply higher energy costs for fresh produce.

In 1999, the cost of TFP foods for the "reference family" (men and women aged 20-50y with 2 children aged 6-8 y and 9-11 y) that met food guide pyramid guidelines was Rs. 142,800/wk. This cost is equivalent to Rs. 157,650 $person^{-1} \cdot d^{-1}$, the amount of food stamp benefits. France used linear programming to model the composition of the French diet after the imposition of cost constraints. Analyses were based on dietary data for 837 adults that had been collected in an observational study in the Val-de-Marne region.

Nutrient analyses were based on a food-composition table, which was developed by the French National Institute of Health and Medical Research. Estimated national prices for 55 foods-excluding baby foods, rarely consumed foods, and alcohol-were added to the database.

The prices were provided by the National Institute of Statistics and Economic Studies and were supplemented with retail prices from super-markets in the Paris area. Linear programming was designed to be consistent with the usual food consumption in France and to minimise any departure from the usual French diet.

The imposition of cost constraints reduced the proportion of energy contributed by fruit, vegetables, meat, and dairy products and increased the proportion of energy contributed by cereals, added fats, and sweets. The resulting diet was identical in composition to that observed among lower-SES groups and contained the least amounts of β-carotene and vitamin C. Consistent with the energy-cost hypothesis, a reduction in diet costs led to diets high in added sugars and fats, as shown in Figure 5.

The cost benefits of nutrition education for food-assistance recipients provides a rare look at diet quality and diet cost. 371 low-income women enrolled in the Expanded Food and Nutrition Education Programme recorded the amount of money spent monthly on food at the time of programme entry and exit. The Expanded Food and Nutrition Education Programme, implemented by state land-grant universities in the United States, is intended to help the nutritional welfare of low-income families.

A saving of Rs. 450-500/m in family food expenditures was associated with a net increase of 300 kcal/d in daily energy intakes and a significantly higher consumption of carbohydrates (43 g/d). The associated increase in fat intake (8 g/d) was not significant. Neither energy density nor added sugar consumption were measured.

OBESITY AND FOOD-ASSISTANCE PROGRAMMES

Studies of diet quality and food assistance generally use regression models to explain the effects of economic and demographic variables, including programme participation and benefit levels, on one or more food consumption variables. For the most part, the dependent variables are intakes of food energy, protein, and selected micronutrients. The results were decidedly mixed. Whereas FSP participation had positive and significant effects on the consumption of some foods, other nutrient needs were not always met.

Few low-income households meet the twin objectives of spending less than the TFP amount and buying foods that contribute to a healthful diet. Those few people that did meet these objectives spent a larger share of the food dollar on grains, fruits, vegetables, and milk and less on meat, soft drinks, sweets, fats, and alcohol. However, according to USDA surveys, most low-income respondents spent their limited food dollars on energy-dense foods that were largely composed of added sugars and fat.

Studies that used more global measures of diet quality were more successful in showing the benefits of the FSP or the Supplementary Nutrition Programme for Women Infants and Children (WIC). These studies found that the consumption of the 5 main food guide pyramid food groups (ie, those other than fats and sweets) increased as incomes increased.

Studies conducted by the Center for Nutrition Policy and Promotion using 1989-1991 CSFII data found that WIC participation and, to a lesser extent, the FSP were associated with higher-quality diets, as indexed by HEI scores. Otherwise, little is known about the effects of food-assistance programmes on diet quality and dietary energy density. Another research gap concerns measures of acceptance for individual foods and participant satisfaction with the overall quality of the diet. Such information would be useful in tracking satisfaction with food choices provided or recommended by food-assistance programmes.

Food choices and energy intakes in obesity have been explained in terms of biology, physiology, and behaviour. The biological explanation has been that taste preferences or "cravings" for sweet and high-fat foods are driven by central metabolic events, such as serotonin imbalance, altered concentrations of leptin or neuropeptide Y, or the endogenous opiate peptide system. Physiologic explanations have invoked the glycemic index of foods, insulin resistance, and adipose tissue metabolism.

Psychological explanations have addressed inadequate nutrition knowledge, excessive vulnerability to the external environment, addictive personality, and the consumption of high-fat foods in search of comfort. Environmental approaches have blamed the wide availability of snacks, fast foods, and soft drinks; the presence of vending machines in schools; and the phenomenon of "supersising" of fast foods eaten outside the home.

Television advertising has been cited as a factor contributing to higher energy and fat intakes and so has the marketing of energy-dense foods. In 1997, food manufacturers, food retailers, and food services reportedly spent US $11 billion on advertising, much of it on foods containing added sugars and fat. Studies suggest that some of this advertising may be targeted at children and at low-income consumers.

As indicated above, such foods provide energy at a much lower cost than do fresh vegetables and fruit, which are perceived as luxury items and are not always easily accessible. Growing portion sizes are another example of how the food industry provides inexpensive extra energy at lower unit cost.

The most commonly cited examples of supersizing tend to involve foods composed of refined grains, added sugars, and fat. The notion of the economic costs of obesity invariably refers to the costs of obesity and related diseases to society. There has been little emphasis on the low economic costs of becoming obese. At world market prices, the cost of refined sugar is ≈10 cents/lb (454 g). In other words, close to 80 000 kJ can be purchased for Rs.1.

The current economic hypothesis is that high energy intakes, not only in the United States but worldwide, may be driven by the very low cost and reinforced by positive hedonic properties of energy-dense foods. Obesity has been linked with the excessive consumption of both sugars and fats. Whether fat as opposed to sugar consumption is to blame is a controversial issue.

Some researchers believe that excessive carbohydrate, as opposed to fat, consumption is responsible for the current obesity epidemic. This argument rests on the observation that the percentage of energy from fat decreased from 38% to 34% between 1976-1980 and 1988-1991, whereas the prevalence of obesity increased.

In reality, both incomes and total fat consumption (in g/d) have continued to increase, as have total energy intakes. One mechanism to hold down diet costs is to increase the energy-density of the diet through the consumption of more grains and added sugars and fats. Obesity rates increase as energy intakes increase, but food spending (as a percentage of income) decreases disproportionately relative to spending on other goods.

Consumer food choices are driven by taste, cost, and convenience, and to a lesser extent by health and variety Research has linked growing obesity rates with a growing consumption of snacks, fast foods, and soft drinks (1-9) and with the consumption of high-energy-density diets. What energy- dense foods have in common is low energy cost, due in part to the presence of added sugars and fat.

Some nutrition professionals have already noted that diets consumed by groups with a lower SES provide cheap, concentrated energy from fat, sugar, cereals, potatoes, and meat products but very little intake of vegetables, fruits, and whole grains. Yet any discussion of dietary energy density in relation to diet costs has been missing from the mainstream literature on the determinants of obesity in the United States.

Economic resources may shift dietary choices toward an energy-dense, highly palatable diet that provides maximum calories per the least volume and the least cost. The hypothesis that healthier diets may indeed cost more has many policy implications. One issue is whether economic incentives can promote healthful eating more effectively than do current strategies, on the basis of theoretical models for behavioural change. The USDA has linked a lower consumption of added sugars among WIC participants to the provision of WIC-supplied juices and cereals.

There are also studies on price supports for vegetables and fruit and on the manipulation of snack prices in vending machines to encourage the consumption of lower-fat items. If this economic approach is to be successful, we need a better understanding of how food prices affect consumer food choices and the selection of a healthy diet.

Reducing the energy density of the diet is a worthy objective; the question is, can it be achieved without simultaneously increasing the cost and reducing the palatability of the diet? If long-term compliance with recommended diets is to be achieved by persons with a limited food budget, the foods must be affordable and acceptable. More work is needed to explore strategies for systematically shifting taste and food preferences in the direction of less energy-dense foods. A shift to a diet with a greater emphasis on fruit, vegetables, and whole grains would be consistent with the gradual change in consumption from full- to reduced-fat dairy products seen over the past 30 years.

The current focus of obesity research has been on environmental factors that promote inactive lifestyles and excess energy intakes. The present economic approach suggests that food choices and diet quality are influenced by social and economic resources and by food costs. Low-cost, energy-dense diets are likely to contain added sugars and vegetable fats. Such diets have been and will continue to be associated with obesity and overweight.

However, the relevant features of obesity promoting diets may not be the percentage of energy from sugar or fat but rather high palatability and low energy cost. These issues are inextricably linked to agricultural commodity prices, imports, tariffs, and trade. Americans are gaining more and more weight while consuming more added sugars and fats and are spending a lower proportion of their income on food. No longer a purely medical issue, obesity has become a societal and public health problem.

11

ECONOMICS OF FOOD LABELLING

Designing a labelling policy to achieve a social objective like a healthier population highlights some of the problems at the heart of any government decision to intervene in labelling, for whatever reason. As with any policy, the costs and benefits of government intervention in labelling must be weighed, and the sometimes conflicting demands of economic efficiency, consumer and producer concerns, public opinion, political expediency, and current events must be sorted and evaluated.

There is a lot to know about the food we eat. For example, the ingredients for a jar of spaghetti sauce, a box of cereal, or a cup of coffee could come from around the corner or around the world; they could be grown with numerous pesticides or just a few; they could be grown on huge corporate organic farms or on small family-run conventional farms; they could be harvested by children or by machines; they could be stored in hygienic or pest-infested storage facilities; or they could increase or decrease the risk of cancer.

A description of any one food product could include information on a myriad of attributes. Consumers, food processors, third-party entities, and governments all play a role in determining which of a food's many attributes are described on food labels. Consumers use their purchasing power (their consumption choices) and political activities to help determine which attributes are described on labels. Private firms seek out attributes that are attractive to consumers and voluntarily provide information about these attributes when the benefits of doing so outweigh the costs.

Third-party entities, including private organisations, governments, and international organisations, contribute to enhancing the intelligibility and credibility of information about some food attributes through standard setting, certification, and enforcement. These services can increase the amount of information supplied by labels.

Information on some attributes be included on food labels. Government intervention in labelling in the United States has served three main purposes: *to ensure fair competition among producers, to increase consumers' access to information, and to reduce risks to individual consumer safety and health.*

DECISION OF VOLUNTARY LABELLING

For a firm, labelling is one of many advertising options and its labelling decision can be examined just like any other advertising decision. Assuming that firms attempt to maximise profits, they will add more information to product packaging so long as each additional message generates more revenues than it costs.

A label is intended to help consumers differentiate the labelled product from otherwise similar products. A label calls to consumers' attention the desirable attributes of the product. When a firm labels its product, it assumes that the information it provides is important to consumers and that they will respond by changing their purchase decisions.

The incentive for firms to advertise, claiming that if a firm's advertising has any effect, it will be to allow the firm to sell more without reducing the price it charges or to raise the price without losing sales or market share. While it is easy to say that firms disclose information that is advantageous to them, deciding which attributes consumers will find desirable is not a trivial problem.

If firms could easily decide which information is advantageous to disclose on labels and how to disclose it, big Madison Avenue advertising firms would be neither big nor located on Madison Avenue. The labelling decision is complex for two reasons.

First, for even the simplest of products, there are many attributes that could be labelled. For example, the attributes of bottled water include the size and shape of container, trace mineral content, and place of origin. Some bottled-water labels name particular springs or types of springs while others suggest snow-melt from Alpine mountains as a source. **Second**, the labelling decision is complex because consumers are not all alike. Consumers have diverse preferences.

Labelling decisions may enhance economic efficiency by helping consumers to target expenditures toward products they most want. Thus, in their drive to persuade the maximum number of consumers to purchase their products, firms may provide a public service by increasing the information available to consumers. The value of this service depends on the importance consumers attach to the attribute and the difficulty they face in assessing the attribute on their own.

Economic studies have characterised product attributes as search, experience, or credence attributes. Search goods are those for which consumers examine product characteristics, such as price, size, and colour, before purchasing. Experience goods are those for which consumers evaluate attributes after purchasing the product. For example, consumers choose particular brands of canned tuna without sampling the product first. Credence goods have attributes that consumers cannot evaluate even in use.

For example, consumers cannot inspect particular produce items and determine whether they were grown organically or whether they are the result of biotechnology. Consumers cannot inspect canned tuna and determine if the tuna was caught without harming dolphins. Though producers may wish to conceal the negative attributes of their products, a number of factors make this difficult, even for experience and credence goods. First, consumer skepticism may lead to a situation in which consumers are informed about all attributes of goods.

For example, if a consumer could not determine the contents of a box before purchase and had to rely on a label claiming that the box contained "at least three oranges," a rational consumer might assume exactly three oranges. If there were really four oranges in the box, the seller would say so because a box of four would command a higher price than a box of three. So if the rational consumer expects the worst-that labels are as optimistic as truth permits-the firm has an incentive to highlight all the positive attributes of its product.

Consumers can infer that every attribute that the firm does not discuss is negative; either the product does not possess desirable attributes or attributes are of low quality. Second, warranties offer consumers a mechanism for deducing product information for credence goods. If a product has an observable characteristic related to the credence attributes, the firm can offer a warranty. For example, suppose an automobile manufacturer wanted to distinguish its product from other cars with a claim of overall better quality. While it is difficult to observe the quality of a car, a low-quality car will break down more often than a high-quality car.

An automobile dealer can offer a warranty against particular types of failures. Unwillingness to offer warranties for particular failures amounts, in the eyes of skeptical consumers, to admission that some attributes of the car are low quality. Third, competition among firms also reinforces consumers' ability to deduce relatively complete information about the hidden quality dimensions of products. For example, the producer of a food product low in fat might voluntarily advertise that fact.

A competitor with a similar product low in both fat and sodium would have an incentive to advertise its product's two desirable attributes. Consumers would then be suspicious of products that failed to make both claims. This competitive disclosure, which Ippolito and Mathios named the "unfolding" theory, results in explicit claims for all positive aspects of products and allows consumers to make appropriate inferences about foods without claims.

The unfolding theory also leads to the conclusion that firms' advertising would inadvertently alert consumers to negative aspects of products. For example, without any cigarette labelling requirements, the cigarette brand that advertises less tar would be alerting consumers to a negative aspect of all cigarettes. Disclosure of tar levels would be likely among low-tar cigarettes and nonexistent among others. The unfolding theory implies that the presence of advertising is a signal of quality and that competitive products without such advertising are alerting consumers to its absence.

Empirical tests of the effectiveness of the market in producing full disclosure of quality to consumers have yielded mixed results. When the NLEA went into effect, nutrition labelling was provided on a voluntary basis. The frequency with which food products carried nutrition labels in 1992-93, found that for food groups defined as salted snacks, cereal, yogurt, and margarine spreads, almost all products carried voluntary nutrition labels, regardless of nutrition profiles.

Market Incentives

While consumer skepticism, warranties, and competition among firms may expose many product attributes, they are not always sufficient to guarantee complete disclosure. For example, when an entire product category has an undesirable characteristic that cannot be changed appreciably, unfolding depends on producers of entirely different foods to draw attention to the undesirable characteristics. In these cases unfolding may be weaker than in cases where variations exist within the same product category.

Another limitation to market incentives to disclose information arises when information has a "public good" aspect, that is when information pertains to a whole product type, not one particular product. In these cases, even if information increases sales, the chances that the benefits of labelling outweigh the costs for a single firm are reduced: the costs are borne by the single firms while the benefits are shared by many.

For example, if the producers of Oat Snappy Cereal label their cereal boxes with the information that oat bran cereals have been linked to lower heart disease, they provide information not only about their cereal, but also about all other oat cereals as well. In this case, the information is a public good, and like all public goods is less likely to be produced voluntarily. Market incentives and legal prohibitions may also be unable to eliminate partial disclosure and innuendo. The possibility of deception erodes the efficiency of the market. Widespread deception makes consumers less responsive to messages, even those that provide truthful information. It makes consumers doubt the veracity of claims made by honest producers.

Third-Party Services

Third-party services could change the private, voluntary labelling decision of firms by either reducing the costs or increasing the benefits of labelling. These services bolster the credibility of voluntary labelling, thereby facilitating market transactions and increasing market efficiency. These services could prove valuable in both domestic and international markets. The primary services that third-party entities offer to help strengthen labelling claims are standard setting, testing, certification, and enforcement.

Standards: Standards establish the level of quality that a good must possess. Standards set by third-party entities facilitate market transactions to the extent that the standards are recognised by numerous producers and consumers. Successful third-party standards establish a common terminology for goods possessing the same quality characteristics.

Without standards, many market transactions would require lengthy negotiation about the quality characteristics of a product. Standards could also establish the way that labelled information is presented, ensuring that information is provided in a uniform manner, allowing consumers to compare products more easily.

Testing services: Third-party testing services help producers strengthen their claims of product quality by providing a more objective measure of product attributes. Particularly for credence attributes, testing services increase the value of the information provided by the label. In addition, third-party testing services could reduce the costs of verifying that standards have been met.

If the average cost of testing declines with the volume of tests run, it may be less expensive for one party to provide testing for many firms rather than for each firm to test or for each consumer to try to test the veracity of product claims. In some cases, testing is not possible and identity-preservation systems, in which product quality is assured by strict segregation and tracking systems, may emerge.

Certification: Third-party certification provides assurances to consumers that the information supplied by firms is correct. Consumers may question the validity of the information provided by firms, particularly for credence goods. Third-party certification provides consumers with an objective evaluation of the product's quality attributes and helps firms establish credible market claims. Third-party certification could also be used to establish the credentials of other third-party services, including other third-party certifiers. Accreditation is a process for certifying certifiers.

Enforcement: Third-party enforcement of quality standards provides further assurances that quality claims are valid. If firms making fraudulent claims are penalised, incentives to make truthful claims are strengthened. The more onerous the penalty for fraud and the higher the probability of being caught, the more reliable quality claims are likely to be. Third-party enforcement services include watch-dog services, de-certification, and legal requisites.

Watch-dog-type enforcement services rely on negative publicity to discourage fraud. Firms with valuable reputations will be most susceptible to this type of enforcement. De-certification provides a clear indication that a product has failed to comply with quality standards and represents the most powerful enforcement tool available to most private third-party certifiers. Decertification by government entities could carry the added penalty of prohibiting marketing of the product. Legal requisites concerning advertising provide the ultimate enforcement against fraudulent quality claims, even for voluntary claims.

Third-party services can be provided by a wide variety of entities, including consumer groups, producer associations, private third-party entities, national governments, and international organisations. For example, the Good Housekeeping Institute, founded for the purpose of consumer education and product evaluation, sets product standards and provides consumer guarantees for a wide range of goods including foods; a nonprofit membership organisation, facilitates development of voluntary private-sector standards for a wide range of products; Underwriters Laboratories (UL), a private nonprofit entity, provides standards and certification, primarily for electrical appliances; the Council of Better Business Bureaus works with the National Advertising Review Board to investigate questions of truth and accuracy in national commercial advertising; the USDA's Agricultural Marketing Service (AMS) has established standards for 233 agricultural commodities; and ISO, a worldwide federation of national standards bodies, promotes the development of standardisation and international standards for a wide range of products.

Producers could employ just one or two labelling services, or they could employ a combination of the four. For any branch along the labelling services tree, the government provides an ultimate enforcement: fraud is always subject to legal sanctions. Even with private standards and private testing and certification, the government, through laws prohibiting fraudulent and deceptive advertising, plays a role in enforcing the truthfulness of product claims.

The first-branch of the labelling tree shows the case where a private third-party entity sets standards, provides testing and certification, and enforces truthful compliance with standards. There are many examples of this case, including most kosher labelling and private organic standards. The second-branch of the tree illustrates the case where private entities set standards, and provide certification and enforcement, but the government assists in the process by providing testing services or accreditation of testing services.

Such a situation could emerge when standards are technically difficult to test for and government services help establish testing norms. For example, USDA's Grain Inspection, Packers and Stockyards Administration (GIPSA) has established a reference laboratory to evaluate and verify the validity of analytical techniques applied to the detection of genetically enhanced traits in grains and grain products. The third-branch of the tree illustrates the case where the government sets voluntary quality standards and provides for protection against fraud, but relies on private testers and certifiers to guarantee that standards have been met.

In some cases, the voluntary standards set by AMS are certified and enforced by private entities. The fourth-branch of the labelling tree shows the case where the government is responsible for providing or accrediting providers of all four services. For example, many States set standards for organic foods and provide certification and enforcement services. In general, the value of the labelling service depends on the credibility and reputation of the entity providing the service. Services provided by entities that are trusted and well known by a large number of consumers will be most successful in reducing search and information costs, facilitating market transactions, and increasing market efficiency. In many cases, national governments or associations of national governments may be the most widely recognised and reputable third-party providers of labelling servces.

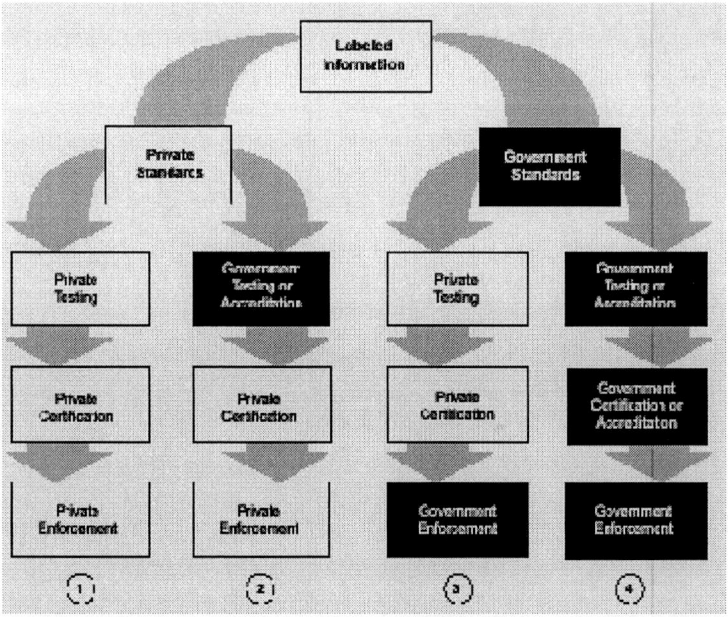

Figure 1: Labelling tree

The value of third-party labelling services also depends on the extent to which they are responsive to consumer preferences and technological capabilities. This is particularly true for standards. If standards are more lenient or strict than consumer preferences, consumers will search out goods with quality standards that match their preferences more closely.

For example, if standards are so strict that production costs rise beyond consumers' willingness to pay, consumers will seek products with lower standards. If standards surpass the technological ability of producers to meet or of consumers to verify, they will eventually lose their value. For example, a standard that sets a zero tolerance level for biotech ingredients in non-biotech oils would be virtually impossible to verify given the current state of biotech testing.

Neither consumers nor producers would be able to test compliance, and the standard would become meaningless. The most flexible standards with respect to changes in consumer preferences or technology may actually be those set without third-party participation. In the absence of third-party standards, producers and consumers must establish standards and quality requirements through contractual agreements-most of which are updated periodically to reflect changes in consumer preferences and technologies.

Standards set by government or international organisations may often be the least flexible and most difficult to modify in response to changes in preferences and technologies. This prohibition was not considered overly restrictive when it was written into law in the 1950's. However, since then, chemical detection sensitivity has increased by several orders of magnitude, and carcinogens have been detected in foods once considered hazard free. Standards can also be misused, as when they are used to establish barriers to entry benefiting a particular, usually well-established group of producers.

Such standards not only suppress fair competition, they hinder innovation and technological change. These standards are costly to consumers and to market development. If properly designed and implemented, third-party standard setting, testing, certification, and enforcement all increase the value of a label by increasing the reliability and credibility of the labelling claim. These services reduce uncertainty for producers, reduce search and information costs for consumers, and increase the likelihood that consumers will purchase those goods and services that best match their preferences. Because they increase the value of information, these third-party services can increase the amount of information that producers choose to provide to consumers through product labels.

These services can enhance the efficiency of domestic and international markets. Though potentially very valuable, third-party services can work only with producer incentives. These services cannot change producers' fundamental reluctance to disclose information about undesirable product characteristics. Other mechanisms must be employed to encourage disclosure of important negative product attributes.

MANDATORY LABELLING

In addition to a potential role in bolstering voluntary labelling, the government may also decide that some information must be labelled. Most demands for mandatory labelling (including the "consumer's right to know" and calls for fair competition) arise in two general economic situations: when the market does not supply enough information to allow consumers to make consumption choices mirroring their individual preferences (asymmetric or missing information); and when individual consumption decisions affect social welfare differently than they affect the individual consumer's welfare (externality problems). In both of these situations, social costs and benefits may suggest a different labelling outcome than the one resulting from a private firm's labelling decision.

Correct Asymmetric Information

Properly functioning markets provide a valuable service

to society. In properly functioning markets, consumers are able to purchase the goods and services that best match their preferences. As a result, society's resources are used in ways that match consumers' preferences. However, sometimes the market supplies too little information to enable consumers to make consumption choices reflecting their preferences.

One such situation occurs when there is asymmetric information, that is, the seller knows relevant information about a product that the buyer does not know. In cases of asymmetric information, resources are used less efficiently than with perfect, symmetric information. Asymmetric information may particularly be a problem in markets for foods with negative credence attributes or for markets in which information has a public good aspect. In these cases, firms may have no incentive to provide consumers with information.

As a result, consumers may end up purchasing goods that do not match their preferences. In this case, the market does not work efficiently: goods that would be profitable with full disclosure may go unproduced while those of lesser value to consumers are produced instead. In some cases of asymmetric information, the government may decide to intervene in the market to require producers to disclose critical information.

Mandatory labels targeting asymmetric information are designed to provide consumers with greater access to information and to increase the efficiency of the market. The objective of government intervention in these types of cases is not so much to alter consumption behaviour but to increase informed consumption. Another type of information problem that may occur in food markets is that of imperfect information. Unlike the case of asymmetric information, where producers know relevant information about the product that consumers do not, in cases of imperfect or missing information, relevant market information does not exist or is contradictory.

This situation could arise when the long-term health effects of a food or food attributes are unknown, or when scientific opinions differ about the health consequences of consumption. In these cases, the government might require full disclosure of even preliminary or contradictory information to provide consumers with the fullest information possible. It is a perversion of the intent of information provision to wait until full knowledge is available before labelling products. Indeed, if such information is valuable to consumers, it could improve market efficiency as in the case of asymmetric information.

Individual food consumption decisions can have a wide variety of social welfare consequences, including effects on the environment, health and productivity, labour conditions, and farm and industry structure. For example, consumers who choose diets high in saturated fat increase their risk of heart disease and cancer, creating costs not just for themselves, but also for employers and public health systems. Conversely, diets high in oat bran may lower the risk of heart disease, creating productivity gains and medical-care savings that benefit the whole society.

When the food consumption choices of consumers affect the welfare of others, and these welfare effects are not priced, then consumers may consume more or less than is socially optimal. If the price of the food were changed to fully reflect these welfare effects, then the market outcome would be socially optimal. For example, if the price of saturated fat were raised to reflect the costs of public health impacts, then less saturated fat would be consumed. Economists describe situations in which action of one economic agent affects the utility or production possibilities of another in a way that is not reflected in the market-place as externalities.

Where private consumption decisions result in externalities, social welfare may be maximised by a labelling choice that differs from the one generated by private firms. In the diet example, the potential social benefits of providing dietary information on labels include a healthier, more productive population and reductions in medical costs. These potential benefits may be larger than the increase in profits that compose a private firm's labelling benefits.

As a result, the social benefits of labelling may outweigh the social costs even though the private benefits do not outweigh private costs. The opposite could also be true, with negative net social benefits and positive net private benefits. For example, the social costs of labelling red wine with the information that moderate consumption lowers the risk of heart disease may be greater than the social benefits.

The potential social costs of such a label include increased rates of birth defects, car accidents, and alcohol-related health costs, while the potential social benefit is the reduction in heart disease. The private firm's costs of redesigning labels are potentially much lower than the benefits of increased sales. In externality cases where private firms do not supply relevant information, the government may decide to intervene in labelling decisions to try to maximise net social benefits.

Government-mandated labelling can be a useful tool for achieving social objectives because of the potential power of information to influence consumption decisions. The primary difficulty in regulating to achieve a social objective comes in clearly identifying "the social objective." Although particular special or public interest groups may advocate labelling as a means of influencing consumption decisions to align them with a particular social objective, such objectives may not be widely valued.

Society is composed of a diverse variety of individuals and interest groups. It is not a trivial task to design regulation that truly reflects widespread public interest. This is not to say that it is difficult to identify activities that affect social welfare. In fact, if social welfare is defined to include the "public purse," it may be difficult to find an activity that does not qualify. What is difficult is determining if the benefits of a given social objective merit the costs of government intervention in the market.

Even if informational and social welfare considerations indicate that there may be a role for government intervention, labelling may not be an effective policy tool. Information policy such as labelling generally is not very effective and there are some circumstances, such as when people do not read or do not care about the information on the label, in which it may not be effective at all. Empirical studies have found labels to be both successful and unsuccessful in educating consumers and changing consumption behaviour. These and other studies highlight the observation that consumers often make hasty food choices in grocery stores and usually do not scrutinise food labels.

The format and context of the information are important elements in maximising the possibility that labelled information will influence its audience. Consumers are more likely to read and understand labels that are clear and concise. A large number of warnings or a large list of detailed product information may cause many consumers to disregard the label completely. Even if consumers do consider each piece of information on a label, they may find it difficult to order the information according to importance.

For example, out of 10 warnings on a label, consumers

may have difficulty picking out the most important. As a result, consumers may underreact to important information or over-react to less important information. While clear, concise labels could possibly be designed to address problems of asymmetric information, problems for which information exists, it is unlikely that labels would be successful in addressing problems of imperfect information.

By definition, the information available in these situations is unclear. Not only is it difficult to convey such information on a label, it is difficult for consumers to decipher it. Consumers have a particularly difficult time making sense of small probabilities or of information about an issue that lacks scientific or political consensus. It is unreasonable to expect individuals to process information that has confounded the experts. Providing information that leaves consumers confounded is unlikely to lead to improvements in market efficiency.

A more comprehensive and better targeted approach to inadequate information might include research and science education programmes that stress the probabilistic nature of scientific knowledge. It is important to recognise that informing people, whether by labels, package inserts, or more extensive programmes, is but part of the larger problem of helping people cope with the risks and uncertainties of modern life. Labels may also be a poor means of addressing problems of externalities and advancing social objectives.

Individuals tend to weigh their individual private costs and benefits, exclusive of externality costs, when making consumption decisions. Even if certain individuals alter their behaviour to completely reflect externality costs, the fact that others do not means that the objective will probably not be met. For example, while some consumers may purchase only free-range chickens, the goal of more humane treatment of chickens will not be achieved so long as most consumers continue to purchase coop chickens. Differing preferences for the targeted consumption good may also lead to less than optimum results. For example, even if all agree that a slimmer, fitter population is a good social (and personal) objective, some consumers' preferences for fatty foods and inactivity may outweigh their valuation of the social objective.

Labels may also be unable to change behaviour enough to meet a social objective if some consumers free-ride on others' socially responsible behaviour. For example, although a consumer may feel that sea turtles should be protected and that strict laws protecting them should be enforced, he or she may decide that eating one small bowl of turtle soup will not really make a difference. The uneven distribution of collective benefits also mitigates against the achievement of social goals through labelling.

Even if individuals have similar preferences over the social outcome, the fact that some benefit more than others probably means that not everyone will change their behaviour to match the social optimum. Economic theory identifies a number of policy tools that may be more suited to redressing externalities than information remedies. Bans, quotas, production regulations or standards, and Pigouvian taxes may all be more successful than mandatory labels in adjusting consumption and production to better match socially optimum levels.

Regardless of the objective, effective labelling hinges on the existence of standards, testing, certification, and enforcement services. To establish credible, effective mandatory labelling, the government must ensure that every step along the labelling tree (fig. 1) exists. The government must ensure that the quality standards in questions are clear and achievable; that testing services, if necessary, are available to measure the validity of labelling claims; that producers (and consumers) are able to certify or otherwise prove the validity of the quality claim; and that a mechanism for enforcing labelling rules exists, including a mechanism to punish producers who make fraudulent claims. The government must either perform these services or accredit third-party agents to perform them. Mandatory labelling laws that are not supported by standards, testing, certification, and enforcement services could result in confusion and actually increase transaction costs.

Costs and Benefits

Effective labelling may generate a variety of benefits. Effective or not, it generates a variety of costs. Policy-makers must weigh the benefits and costs of labelling as well as the distribution of benefits and costs to determine whether labelling is an appropriate policy option.

Measuring the Benefits of Mandatory Labelling: In measuring the benefits of mandatory labelling, analysts must consider a wide set of effects, few of which are found on a balance sheet. The task of actually measuring benefits may involve difficult methodological and philosophical problems.

The primary benefits of a government labelling programmes are increases in informed consumption and socially desirable changes in consumption behaviour. The fact that these outcomes usually involve goods without established market prices, such as health and environmental quality, makes it particularly difficult to assign dollar amounts to these outcomes for cost-benefit comparisons. The fact that the stated objective often involves social goals over which different groups of consumers may have diametrically opposing opinions and valuations makes the task of measuring benefits even more challenging.

Another type of benefit arising from government intervention in labelling could be those stemming from product reformulation. Firms that are forced to disclose negative characteristics of their products may choose to reformulate to eliminate the negative characteristics rather than risk losing sales as a result of the disclosure label. In this way, labelling benefits all consumers who use the products, not just those who read the label.

These benefits could actually be quite large. Health claims on cereal boxes helped change consumer behaviour and resulted in significant product innovation. Some analysts argue that more healthful foods resulting from reformulation may be the largest benefit of labelling. Social benefits other than those targeted by the labelling policy may also arise from government-mandated labelling.

Cost-benefit analyses of labelling policies should include the value of such policies in (1) generating consumer confidence in product quality; (2) establishing the parameters for advertising; (3) signaling which of the product's quality attributes are important; and (4) reinforcing other forms of education at the consumer level.

Measuring the Costs of Mandatory Labelling: The costs of government labelling policy could be as far ranging and difficult to measure as the benefits. The least difficult costs to gauge are the actual costs to the government of programme initiation, administration, and enforcement. Industry costs of relabelling are also relatively easy to assess and, in some cases, these costs may be absorbed in the normal label-change cycle if the compliance period is sufficiently long.

Some of the industry costs of labelling will most

likely be passed on to consumers in higher prices. As a result, consumers who do not particularly value the information are forced to pay for it through higher prices. A redistribution of welfare occurs. The costs of any reformulation resulting from labelling laws could also be quite large-and quite difficult to measure. Labelling programmes may also result in changes to industry structure that could be viewed as costs. For example, mandatory labelling could result in higher additional per-unit costs for small firms than for large firms.

As a result, the market price may not compensate small firms for the additional costs of labelling, thus putting them at a competitive disadvantage. This could impose disproportionate costs on rural economies and communities. Costs of additional labelling also include the extent to which it dilutes the effectiveness of the information already included on the product label. As mentioned before, too much information on a label reduces the chances that consumers will read it.

If consumers do read it, too much information reduces the chance that they will be able to accurately evaluate the importance of each piece of information. The distribution of the benefits and costs of labelling could play as important a role in influencing the government's decision to intervene in labelling as the overall level of net benefits. Any intervention will yield some distributional consequences.

Changes in consumption choices or product reformulation resulting from labelling will lead to growth in some sectors of the economy and declines in others. Policy that imposes costs on certain critical groups, even if it confers benefits on a wide variety of other groups, may be undesirable from a political or equity standpoint.

NUTRITION LABELLING

Nutrition labels are intended to help consumers choose more healthful foods. Providing nutrition information increases incentives for producers to create more healthful foods and aids consumers in choosing a healthier diet, which leads to lower costs from dietrelated illnesses. In contrast to nutrition "standards," nutrition labels do not constrain choice, they allow consumers to balance their own nutritional preferences and requirements. The costs of mandatory food labelling include higher production costs and food prices.

The health benefits of nutrition labelling are difficult to measure and in many cases have been obscured by other factors that affect health, such as lack of exercise, increased food consumption, and increased consumption of ready-to-eat foods. The benefits of mandatory nutrition labelling appear to exceed the costs.

Producers will decide to include a nutrition label if sales revenues will rise by more than the cost of the label. FDA estimated 61 percent of annual sales of packaged foods had nutrition labels in 1988. This translated into approximately 40 percent of all brands, so for many producers the private benefits of nutrition labels exceeded the costs. Some information is revealed by a firm's decision not to provide a label. For example, the lack of an organic label tells the consumer the food is not organic as clearly as would a label saying "not organic." However, this unfolding process is not as robust for nutritional content because of the complexity of nutrition information. Therefore, the producer's decision not to include a nutrition label may convey little information for consumers.

Nutrition labels are less beneficial if consumers have difficulty using them. A third-party service, in this case the Federal Government, had the potential to increase the benefits of nutrition labels by standardising the label. Standards created by the government dictate the format of the label, the list of micro and macronutrients that should appear on the label, serving sizes, location of the label, and units of measurement. This standard aids consumers in making comparisons between products and in interpreting nutrition information.

That the private market failed to provide nutrition information is not alone sufficient to justify mandatory nutrition labels. For society to be better off with mandatory nutrition labels, the social benefits of labelling must exceed the costs. FDA attempted to discover if the social costs or benefits were greater in the economic analysis of the proposed amendment to the nutrition labelling regulations. FDA based the estimate of benefits on health improvements resulting from consumers' changing their diets in response to the nutrition information. The health benefits arising from the labelling changes were assessed using a three-step model:

a) Changes in consumer diets, leading to,
b) Changes in health states, and
c) Valuation of these health changes.

The analysis focused on changes in consumption of fat and cholesterol and their effect on cancer and coronary heart disease (CHD). The first step of the model, changes in consumer behavior, hinged on how much consumers would change their diets based on the newly available nutrition information. To approximate the amount of the change, the FDA looked at a small study that measured how consumers changed their consumption of fat and cholesterol in response to nutrition information flags on grocery store shelves.

Fat consumption fell an average of 1.25 percent and cholesterol an average of 0.1 percent for consumers at that grocery store. This change in fat and cholesterol consumption was hypothesised, in turn, to lead to reduced incidence of cancer and CHD. FDA estimated that the decrease in fat and cholesterol due to the nutrition information would prevent 35,179 cancer cases, 4,024 cases of CHD, and 12,902 premature deaths over 20 years. Finally, to estimate the benefits of nutrition labelling, the agency valued this reduction in deaths and illnesses.

Economists attempt to measure consumers' own value of reductions in illnesses and deaths by looking at consumers' willingness to pay for accepting small changes in the probability of death. For example, the wage premium to workers in risky jobs or consumer purchases of safety equipment represents implicit valuation of small probabilities of death. The willingness to pay for the reduction in illnesses and deaths brought about by nutrition labelling was Rs. 162 billion and the reduced medical costs were Rs. 27 billion over 20 years. This Rs.189 billion may underestimate total social benefits. The analysis includes only cancer and CHD.

Many other illnesses are diet related, such as diabetes, arthritis, and stroke. By excluding these other diseases, the analysis underestimates benefits. Also, consumers may value having nutrition information, even if they do not act on it. Other policy tools targeted at improving nutrition, such as nutrition standards, do not provide the flexibility of nutrition labelling. For example, a nutrition standard limiting the amount of salt in a food would constrain all consumers' choices, not just those of consumers on low-salt diets. Consumers have different nutritional needs and concerns. What is a positive nutrition attribute for one consumer may be a negative attribute for another.

For example, a consumer on a low-fat, low-carbohydrate diet may have different definitions of "good" and "bad" foods than one on a high-protein diet. A consumer on a low-carbohydrate, high-protein diet might find low-fat foods that have been formulated by substituting sugar for fat quite undesirable. Labelling is an effective policy tool when consumer preferences and concerns differ. Nutrition labels do not limit choice. By providing more complete, comparable information, standardised nutrition labels may even expand choice.

ORGANIC LABELLING

In the United States, both the private and public (non-Federal) sector provide third-party certification of organic food. Certification standards vary among certifying organisations, and farmers' ability to choose among certifiers varies regionally. The U.S. Department of Agriculture is currently developing regulations that would set national standards for foods marketed as organic and make certification to these standards mandatory for all but the smallest producers.

National standards may reduce transaction costs between farmers and food manufacturers, and may reduce costs of meeting EU organic standards. National standards may help to abate any environmental problems caused by conventional agriculture only to the extent that they increase use of organic farming systems.

Consumers purchase organic products for a variety of reasons: personal safety, which might be compromised by dietary intake of pesticides; environmental concerns, such as the impacts of pesticide use on the environment, groundwater, and wildlife; and farmworker safety. Whatever the reasons, demand for organic foods has translated into a price premium for organic goods.

Organic grains and soybeans command price premiums, and the price gap between organic and conventional widened during the late 1990's for some of these crops. Of course, the cost of producing organic foods is also higher than the cost for conventional food. For organic producers to stay in business, organic premiums must cover differences in farm production practices as well as differences in processing and transportation costs, including segregation costs. The premium also must cover any certification costs.

Farmers, food processors, and other businesses that produce and handle organically grown food certainly have a financial incentive to advertise that information. Organic food is a credence good. Consumers cannot visually distinguish organic food from conventional food. Thus, consumers must rely on labels and other advertising tools for product information. Firms would have no way of acquiring a price premium without labels.

As the demand for organic food has grown from a handful of consumers bargaining directly with farmers to millions of consumers acquiring goods from supermarket shelves as well as market stalls, varying State and private institutions providing third-party verification of label claims evolved. Private organisations, mostly nonprofits, began developing certification standards in the early 1970's as a way to support organic farming and thwart fraud. The first organisation to offer third-party certification,

Third-party certification has been developing as a means to set organic production and handling standards and verify that producers meet these standards, thereby strengthening claims of organic product quality. Most large food processors and grain traders now require certification and many growers have turned to certification as a marketing tool. Certification offers producers additional benefits such as greater marketplace recognition, because of the promotion and consumer education activities of certification organisations, and may facilitate greater information exchange among participating farmers.

However, small producers may currently receive fewer benefits from certification relative to the costs of becoming certified. In California, for example, certification is much more common among large producers than among smaller ones. Most private certifiers charge fees on a sliding scale based on the farmer's gross sales of organic products, number of acres operated, or other measure of size, while State certifying programmes often charge only nominal, unremunerative fees to producers of all sizes.

Even with voluntary certification increasingly available from State and private certifiers, organic food producers and processors experienced a number of marketing problems as the industry expanded in the 1980's, and led the industry request for national organic standards. One problem was that, even though industry standards were largely overlapping, small differences caused disagreements among certifying agents over whose standards would apply to multi-ingredient organic processed products.

The Organic Foods Production Act (OFPA) passed in 1990 largely to address these marketing problems. The OFPA requires the Secretary of Agriculture to establish an organic certification programme for farmers, wild-crop harvesters, and handlers of agricultural products that have been produced using organic methods. **The stated objectives of this legislation are:**

- To establish national standards governing the marketing of certain agricultural products as organically produced products;
- To assure consumers that organically produced products meet a consistent standard; and
- To facilitate interstate commerce in fresh and processed food that is organically produced. This legislation will require that all except the smallest organic growers must be certified by a State or

private agency accredited under national standards currently being developed by USDA.

State and private groups that currently certify growers and processors are expected to seek accreditation by USDA when the national organic standards are implemented. USDA has released two proposed rules to implement this legislation. The most controversial aspects of the first proposal-the potential to allow the use of genetic engineering, irradiation, and sewage sludge in organic production-were dropped from the second proposal.

Also, USDA programme fees were lowered in the second proposal. The second proposal drew only 40,000 comments, many expressing support for the revisions. USDA lacked the data to make a quantitative estimate of the benefits of the proposed rule, or to calculate net benefits, but expects many different groups to benefit. The primary benefits from implementation of the proposed rule are expected to be improved consumer protection from false and misleading claims, and potentially improved access to international markets from elevating reciprocity negotiations to the national level.

The costs of the proposed regulation are the direct costs for accreditation and the costs of complying with the specific standards in the proposal, including the reporting and record-keeping requirements. Certifiers will be charged fees based on the actual costs of the accreditation work done by USDA staff. Smaller certifiers, with less complex programmes, are expected to pay lower fees. Organic farmers, ranchers, and wild-crop harvesters will have to pay fees for organic certification from a State or private certifier, but will not be charged any additional fees by USDA.

One general issue with standards set by government is that they may be less flexible than industry standards, and may reduce innovation. Organic production methods are still developing. If national standards are fixed, certifiers will have less flexibility to promote innovation by setting new standards. In this case, sellers would be unable to communicate their willingness and ability to innovate, and consumers would be unable to signal their preferences, selecting foods with innovative characteristics. On the other hand, food processors and distributors might benefit from holding all certifiers to exactly the same standard.

For example, if most organic food consumers dislike the idea of biotech foods, an organic standard that prohibits biotech means processors and distributors only have to observe the organic label to know that the food they purchase is free of biotech attributes. They would not have to be concerned with the possibility that some certifiers might allow biotech. Thus, any choice for a standard will embody some tradeoffs. Under the current proposal, State and private certifiers are required to have programs that meet the national standard.

State certification programmes would be allowed to have organic standards that are more strict than the national standard, but would not be allowed to block interstate trade of products that meet the national standard. Private certification programmes would not be allowed to set stricter standards, although they could meet contractual arrangements for stricter standards, label additional requirements, and propose changes to the national standard.

Most countries in Europe and several States offer some financial support for conversion to organic farming systems as a way to capture the environmental benefits of these systems. Organic crop production is eligible for cost-share support with Federal conservation funds in Iowa, for example, and in Minnesota, the State will reimburse two-thirds of the cost of organic certification.

Some States that run certifying programmes subsidise programme costs with general revenues.

The Organic Foods Protection Act may also have implications for the structure of the organic farming industry. All certifiers will need to pay for accreditation, and all organic farmers with sales over $225,000 will need to pay for certification to label their products as organic. According to USDA's regulatory impact analysis, even with the small business exemptions, some small organic farms and some small certifiers may exit the industry and small operations may be discouraged from entering the industry.

However, the analysis indicates that other features of the national organic programme, such as the livestock standards, which restrict confinement operations, may be easier for small operations to comply with than for large. The national standard is likely to have only a modest impact on environmental externalities caused by conventional production methods. Organic food is still a niche market in the United States-a small portion of agricultural production requiring only a small portion of agricultural resources.

Thus, the impact of the national standard will be measured by the extent to which it causes the organic market to grow. The national standard could influence the structure of the certifying industry, especially if State agencies continue to subsidise organic agriculture and have flexibility in setting standards. However, if the national standard increases the demand for organic food, the demand for certification will rise as well.

COUNTRY-OF-ORIGIN

A label will not always influence demand enough to make it worth the cost. Market behaviour suggests that the costs of country-of-origin labels for beef and lamb are greater than the benefits. The following example illustrates why any proposed government intervention in labelling decisions ought to arise from a demonstrated market failure.

Firms Producing Beef and Lamb

If consumers are willing to pay extra for the certainty that their meat was produced domestically, and if labelling is relatively inexpensive, there is a financial incentive to make consumers aware of the different product characteristics. Grocers, meatpackers, and farmers would share the increased revenues and have an incentive to voluntarily label. Why is it that grocery items are not ablaze with country-of-origin labels?

The people who are best informed, and who have the greatest incentive to be informed about the costs and benefits of labelling, are grocers, meatpackers, and farmers. Their voluntary use of labels identifying U.S. products is, at most, rare. Their market behaviour suggests that they believe that net benefits of labelling are negative-costs outweigh benefits. There are at least three possible explanations for rarely observing U.S. country-of-origin labels.

Consumers might not care where their food comes from. If country of origin does not influence demand, there is no incentive to label country of origin. That is, domestic beef and lamb producers may not be able to acquire a competitive advantage over importers by alerting consumers to country of origin. Grocers or meatpackers that did provide country-of-origin labels would incur labelling costs but receive no benefit. Some analysts argue that origin does not matter to U.S. consumers.

A bun fabricated from Canadian wheat, and a meat patty composed of lean meat from Australia and fat trimmings from the United States. Current fast-food restaurant advertising does not mention origin. Instead, it emphasises price, portion size, flavour, and promotional toys. Consumers might prefer the imported product. The lack of domestic labels could mean that consumers want to know the origin of meat products, but view the imported product as superior.

In this case, mandatory labelling would only decrease domestic market share. Most imported lamb comes from New Zealand and Australia and is already consumer-ready packaged. Suppliers in both countries have engaged in promotional activities and frequently label their products, highlighting the country of origin. Often, this labelling goes far beyond minimum legal requirements.

Consumers might prefer domestic products, but not enough to cover labelling costs. Even if consumers do favor domestic over imported products, labelling costs may outweigh the benefits from increased demand. Part of the reason benefits are small is that imported muscle cuts are a small fraction of total domestic beef consumption (1-2 percent in recent years). If labels served to exclude a portion of imported beef, the realised price increase would be relatively small in the short run, and most likely zero in the long run. Livestock industries are characterised by production cycles lasting several years.

Full adjustment to any mandated label requirement would likely also take several years. Physical capital required for beef and lamb production and a stock of animals that is fixed in the short run could eventually adjust to maximise profits under new market conditions. Full adjustment is likely to leave no benefits for producers. The consumers who want labels are the only ones who can benefit from labels over the long run.

To see this, suppose labelling made it possible for farmers to earn above-normal returns. These profits would attract new entrants. Absent any barriers to entry, domestic production would expand, bidding market-price down. Under constant returns to scale, new entry would end when production is so large that price returns to its pre-label level. There, above-normal returns would end. Similarly, below-normal returns earned by importers would induce exit until the import price returned to its original level.

The only persistent effect of labels is to offer consumers product characteristics they want. Similarly, ending a requirement for labels would induce exactly the opposite shortrun impacts. Without labels, consumers would no longer be able to distinguish domestically produced beef and lamb from imports, reducing the demand for domestic production. That is, domestic producers would have a strong interest in maintaining the mandate even though they would be operating at normal rates of return. Losing the mandate would be costly in the short run, from their perspective.

Country of origin is a credence attribute. Existing government programmes, as well as wholesale and retail market conditions, suggest that country-of-origin labels on beef and lamb could be credible to consumers. Problems of verification and certification appear not to be significant reasons for the lack of voluntary use of labels.

USDA's Food Safety and Inspection Service (FSIS) is responsible for labels on meat products. FSIS labelling policy allows fresh muscle cuts of beef and lamb to be identified as "U.S. beef" or "U.S. lamb" so long as the statement is truthful. USDA's Agricultural Marketing Service (AMS) offers a voluntary programme to officially certify that livestock, meat, and meat products originate from the United States and are eligible to be labelled as "U.S. beef."

The voluntary programme certifies that livestock and

meat products have been produced from livestock born, raised, slaughtered, and processed in the United States. In effect, USDA has offered to overcome the major stumbling block for labels: verification and certification. To certify U.S. origin, AMS audits production and processing records. Labelling product characteristics is not new to the meat industry. Poultry products have been sold for years under company labels.

For a country-of-origin label to be credible and verifiable, the industries that produce, distribute, and market beef and lamb would have to undertake some new activities. If they continue to sell both domestic and imported products, they would have to segregate domestic and imported products. Segregation is not new to the meat industry.

Slaughter plants currently segregate beef carcasses once they have been graded. Grading programmes result in some labelling claims that follow products through distribution to the retail level. Carcasses generally move through fabrication grouped according to grade, being packaged in boxes or bags that are appropriately labelled.

Livestock producers associations argued that consumers have a right to know where their food is produced and that consumers want to know where their food is produced. Some livestock producers and producer-related associations argued that consumers prefer domestic beef and lamb for a number of reasons: some consumers believe that domestic food is safer, many wish to support domestic farmers, and many wish to support the pesticide, environmental, and worker-protection-laws under which domestic beef and lamb is produced.

The nice feature of the market mechanism is that efficient outcomes usually occur quickly even if all the sellers do not instantly recognise that consumers want products with particular characteristics. If consumers really wanted domestic products, it would take only one grocer to recognise what consumers want. The lines of consumers at the grocery stores that supplied domestic products and the absence of consumers at all other stores would be a strong signal to all other grocers.

Grocery store meat counters would all quickly begin to offer domestic products once one store began profitable discrimination between domestic and imported meat. As grocers asked meatpackers and distributors for domestic products, that demand would be passed back to farmers. Because there are no impediments to voluntary country-of-origin labelling for beef and lamb, the absence of voluntary labels suggests that labels would not lead to different consumer choices.

In addition, the arguments that imported meat is produced under weaker pesticide, environmental, and worker safety laws may not hold. The United States has imported almost all muscle cuts of beef from Canada and almost all muscle cuts of lamb from Australia and New Zealand. These countries enforce their own pesticide, environmental, and worker safety laws.

There is a reason that markets do not yield efficient outcomes, there is no way to argue that social costs and benefits differ from their private counterparts. The private sector's choices can be assumed to be best. However, even if labels had the effect domestic producers desire, and if imports were produced under weaker pesticide, environmental, and worker safety laws, labels would not solve the problems cited by the livestock producers.

Because beef and lamb, like most agricultural commodities, are exchanged in international markets, the meat excluded from the United States would be sold elsewhere. Other policies might be more effective at redressing international pesticide, environmental, and worker safety problems.

BIOTECH LABELLING

The biotech labelling example illustrates three observations. **First**, to establish successful mandatory labelling requirements, the Government must provide or arrange for standards, testing, certification, and enforcement. **Second**, labelling of complex, unclear information will not reduce information and search costs. **Third**, labelling is not the best policy tool for redressing externalities.

Extensive cultivation of biotech crops began in the United States in the mid-1990's with the introduction of biotech varieties of corn, soyabeans, and cotton. Introduction of these major biotech varieties did not mark the first use of bio-technology in agriculture, but it, along with the use of rbGH in milk production, did herald the widespread introduction of biotech ingredients into a broad variety of food products.

Whether through direct consumption, or by consumption of processed foods or meat, consumers are exposed to a wide variety of food items containing or, in the case of meat, fed with corn, soybeans, or cottonseed meal or oil. The use of biotechnology in flavouring and enzyme production further increases the potential for widespread consumption of food products containing biotech ingredients.

Labelling requirements are established by USDA for meat and poultry and by FDA for all other food products. Both agencies require labelling of a biotech food if the food's composition differs significantly from that of its conventional counterpart. Most biotech foods on the market have been found to be essentially equivalent to their conventional counterparts, hence, most biotech foods are unlabelled. Despite assurances from the government about the safety of biotech foods on the market, some consumers have expressed a desire to be able to distinguish between foods and food products containing biotech ingredients and those that are biotech free.

When deciding whether or not to advertise the non-biotech or biotech characteristics of their products, the question for food producers, including farmers, processors, and manufacturers, is whether someone will eventually compensate them for their trouble. Producers will have the incentive to label and safeguard the integrity of biotech products with positive consumption attributes like better flavour or nutritional content. These characteristics are of value to consumers and advertising their presence may boost demand.

However, most biotech foods currently on the market are "firstgeneration" varieties, varieties with positive producer attributes but no obvious consumer attributes. Producers do not have an incentive to label these products. Currently, the decision confronting most firms is whether to pursue a non-biotech strategy. Such a strategy entails eliminating biotech ingredients from a product, labelling the product as non-biotech, and then marketing the product to consumers who place a value on knowing that their food does not contain biotech ingredients.

Non-Biotech Labelling

Numerous private costs could be incurred in the process of establishing a credible non-biotech product label. First, a producer must consider the opportunity costs associated with the non-biotech labelling decision. The opportunity costs of adopting a non-biotech strategy are the forgone benefits of biotech cultivation and utilisation.

For first-generation biotech crops, these potentially include reduced chemical use, less harmful chemical use, reduced tilling, reduced labor time, less production and financial risk, and in some cases, increased yields.

To date, the evidence on whether or not biotechnology has actually delivered these benefits is positive, although results vary by variety, region, and year.

The economic surplus created by cultivation of biotech varieties is then distributed among farmers, seed producers and biotech firms (higher seed prices, technology fees, and increased profits), and manufacturers and consumers (through lower input prices and food prices). The second set of costs that arises in pursuing a non-biotech marketing strategy are the costs of keeping non-biotech commodities and food products free of biotech material.

This segregation could be achieved by either specialising in biotech or non-biotech, establishing separate facilities for biotech and non-biotech, or taking precautions to sequence or separate biotech and non-biotech production. As an alternative to segregation, processors could choose to reformulate their products to use ingredients from crops that are exclusively non-biotech, thus minimising the risk of inadvertently using a biotech variety.

For example, corn emulsifiers could be replaced with rice emulsifiers. The cost of any of these options varies greatly depending on the flexibility of the production and marketing systems, the tolerance level for biotech content, the volume of biotech and non-biotech commodities and products processed by the system, and the likelihood of achieving economies of scale.

Another set of costs arises in convincing manufacturers and consumers that the product is truly non-biotech. One way to achieve this is to test for biotech content, and a number of private firms have begun to market biotech-testing products. Another method of monitoring the integrity of the non-biotech label is to establish a system of Identity Preservation (IP) in which producers at each stage of the marketing chain attest to the integrity of their non-biotech products.

Such a system relies on strict segregation and product tracking more than on continual testing. Whether they use testing, or IP, or both, it may be difficult for individual firms and farmers to establish a credible non-biotech label. As with other credence goods, consumers may be skeptical of producers' claims. Such skepticism could be fueled by the observation that biotech tests are not completely reliable or consistent, and that it is difficult to ensure the integrity of an IP system.

Benefits to the firm of non-biotech labelling arise to the extent that labelling increases profitability. Labelling could increase a firm's profitability for a number of reasons. **First**, for firms selling biotech food products or commodities that have not been approved for sale in the EU or other foreign markets, pursuing a non-biotech strategy is the only way to gain access to these markets.

For some firms, the benefits of access to these markets could be high, while for others they could be inconsequential. **Second**, firms could profit from a non-biotech label to the extent that such a label enhances the firm's reputation for safety or environmental leadership, thereby strengthening the firm's marketing position. This could be the reason that many baby food manufacturers have adopted a non-biotech strategy. **Third**, the market for biotech foods and commodities is still very unstable and market signals are difficult to decipher.

For example in August 1999, ADM recommended that producers segregate biotech from non-biotech varieties and EU-unapproved from EUapproved varieties, but in February 2000 they withdrew this recommendation. Producers could choose a non-biotech strategy to avoid risk of uncertain biotech markets and to be in a position to gain sales if demand for non-biotech grows.

The **fourth** reason farmers may consider a non-biotech

strategy is that some grain elevators have begun to offer price premiums for non-biotech crops. Evidence suggests that for 1999, premiums ranged from 10-15 cents (roughly a 2-3 percent premium) for soyabeans and from 5-10 cents (roughly a 2-6 percent premium) for corn, though only a small number of elevators offered premiums. The February 2000 survey commissioned by Pioneer Hi-Bred and conducted by Farm Progress Companies estimated that slightly more than 1 out of 10 elevators were planning to offer a price premium for non-biotech products in the fall of 2000.

For some firms, the benefits of creating a non-biotech label outweigh the costs. These firms are tailoring their production to benefit from the emerging markets and potential price premiums for non-biotech products. This is particularly true in the EU where even before labelling was required, many grocery stores and food chains had developed non-biotech product lines. Even in the United States, a number of manufacturers and handlers have moved to create non-biotech product lines, and non-biotech labels can be found in most health food stores.

For other firms, the costs of non-biotech labelling outweigh the benefits. For these firms, the benefits arising from the lower production costs associated with first-generation biotech varieties and a bulk production and marketing system outweigh the benefits of the non-biotech label.

Third-party services could change the labelling decision of many firms by either reducing the costs of biotech labelling or increasing the benefits associated with the non-biotech label. Standards, testing, certification, and enforcement could all facilitate the development of a market for non-biotech foods. Despite the value of third-party services, few are currently available in the United States.

This observation reflects both the small size and youth of the non-biotech market in the United States. It also reflects the difficulty of establishing these services for biotechnology. Third-party entities may have a particularly difficult time establishing well-recognised, achievable standards. Biotech standards or tolerance levels would determine the maximum amount of biotech ingredients allowable in a "non-biotech" commodity or food.

To achieve such standards, the risks of biotech foods would need to be both small and measurable. Like regulation of dietary intake of pesticides, third-party entities could establish biotech tolerances under these conditions. For example, if rodent test results indicated a possibility of harm from biotech foods, analysts could estimate the theoretical risk to humans and use these estimates to guide the setting of tolerance levels. Currently, opinions about biotech risks do not lend themselves to tolerance assessment.

The FDA and many consumers believe that, from a risk perspective, biotech foods and their non-biotech counterparts are identical. That is, there is no additional risk from biotech foods and therefore no reason to set tolerance levels. Some consumer groups, however, characterise the possible outcomes from consuming biotech food as undefinable but catastrophic. On this reasoning, even the smallest amount of biotech food in the food supply should be avoided and therefore, no tolerance granted.

No one is suggesting that there are small risks that might be managed through tolerances. Some national governments are imposing tolerances. In the absence of a consensus on risks, tolerance levels for biotech content are being guided by consumer demand, the feasibility of the system to segregate biotech from non-biotech, and the feasibility of testing technologies to test for biotech content.

The fact that biotech tolerances are currently being determined by rather arbitrary considerations may make it more difficult for government policymakers to participate in setting standards. Policymakers may have particular difficulty reaching consensus on "consumer preferences." In addition, if the government does set standards, there is a danger that these standards could outlive the topical considerations upon which they were based.

It may be difficult for government to change standards in response to changes in consumer preferences and technological advances. Testing for biotech content is another important third-party service, and third-party entities have begun to provide testing services. Two types of tests have been developed to detect use of biotechnology: PCR (polymerase chain reaction) tests and ELISA (enzyme-linked immunosorbent assay) tests. To certify the validity (and limitations) of these tests, private, third-party entities and government both have taken steps to accredit and standardise testing procedures.

The Joint Research Council in the EU has validated both the ELISA and PCR methods. In the United States, the Grain Inspection, Packers and Stockyards Administration (GIPSA) has established a reference laboratory to evaluate and verify the validity of analytical techniques applied to the detection of genetically enhanced traits in grains and grain products.

The third major service that could be supplied by third-party entities is certification. The ultimate viability of a market for non-biotech commodities hinges on the ability of producers to provide credible assurances to consumers that the products they purchase are truly non-biotech. Some third-party certifiers are emerging, many of whom have already established credible identity preservation systems for other types of high-valued commodities and food products such as organic foods.

However, inconsistent standards and variable testing results make certification a risky endeavor. Consistent enforcement of standards, testing, and certification would also decrease transaction costs and increase market efficiency. Again, as with certification, because standards are inconsistent and testing results variable, enforcement may be difficult.

Mandatory labelling will not be effective if it is not accompanied by consistent, achievable standards, testing services (or IP), certification services, and enforcement. In fact, labelling requirements in the absence of these services have more potential to disrupt the market than they do to reduce transaction costs. For example the inconsistent manner in which EU tolerance levels have been applied has increased uncertainty and information and search costs.

In many cases, food manufacturers are uncertain how best to comply with EU standards and ensure access to the European market. Even if the government is able to establish standards, testing (or IP), certification, and enforcement, the effectiveness of biotech labelling for addressing problems of missing or asymmetric information and externality problems is questionable.

A simple label proclaiming "this product contains biotech ingredients" does not convey any information about potential costs and benefits or probabilities. Though such labelling may be informative to some consumers, it may also lead to greater confusion on the part of others and reduce, rather than enhance, economic efficiency. Even if information on theoretical consequences and probabilities were included on the label, it would be unreasonable to expect consumers to be able or willing to evaluate such information.

Labelling is also not the policy tool best suited for reducing any of the potential externalities associated with this technology. Labelling may lead to a better matching of individual consumer preferences, but when preferences differ, some consumers will necessarily be unsatisfied by the social outcome. For example, if consumers perceived biotech foods as posing potential health and environmental risks, then presumably, riskaverse consumers would choose to consume more conventional foods, while the risk-neutral would choose either biotech or conventional foods.

For individual health risks, labels would lead to a better market outcome, allowing consumers to better match their individual health-risk preferences. However, as long as any consumers choose to consume biotech foods, the potential risks to the environment and to public health remain, and the social outcome preferred by biotechaverse consumers is not attained.

For agricultural biotechnology, labelling may be even less successful in correcting for externality problems if the objective is to "internalise" the externality. An externality is internalised when the firm or farmer creating the externality is made to bear the costs of the externality. The cultivation of biotech has the potential to impose externality costs on non-producers, because these producers may need to take precautions to assure that their products are not mixed with biotech products.

For example, non-biotech farmers may need to take precautions to ensure that their crops are not cross-pollinated by biotech crops. Mandatory biotech labelling has been suggested as one means of passing some of these costs back to biotech producers. However, mandatory labelling will probably be unsuccessful in transferring the costs of segregation from non-biotech to biotech producers and consumers.

Even if biotech producers label their products with "may contain biotech" or "does contain biotech," non-biotech producers will still need to certify that their products are indeed non-biotech. As a result, even with mandatory biotech labelling, non-biotech producers and consumers will bear the costs of segregation, and labelling will be unsuccessful at internalising externality costs.

Regulation targeted directly at potential externalities is probably a better policy option than labelling. Biotech cultivation regulations (for example, boundaries and refuges) and well-defined property rights may be better suited to controlling the potential environmental externalities of biotech production.

Once the efficacy of mandatory labelling is established, policy analysts still must determine whether the benefits outweigh the costs. This is a difficult task because most of the social benefits and costs of mandatory labelling are largely theoretical. Labelling advocates cite social benefits ranging from informed consumers to reduced risk of ecological disaster.

Labelling opponents claim that the cost of labelling (and segregation) would be so high that food manufacturers would be forced to stop using biotech crops, thereby reducing the demand for biotech crops to the point that the technology would be abandoned. In this extreme scenario, many of the environmental or social benefits of agricultural biotechnology would be lost. Policy analysts will be hard pressed to calculate the costs and benefits of such theoretical and extreme predictions.

The wide variety of theoretical social costs and benefits, all with varying and unknown probabilities of occurrence, may argue for labelling as one of the best political options for dealing with concerns about biotech consumption and production. Where political or regulatory consensus is not possible, labelling may represent the best compromise solution and the path of least resistance.

Nevertheless, any decision to require labelling must consider whether labelling will have an impact on the social objectives, whether labelling is the least-cost government tool, and of course, whether market forces and individual incentives have already responded to address the policy concern.

■■■

BIBLIOGRAPHY

Boucher PP., (1992) *Cannibal Encounters: Europeans and Island Caribs,* history; cannibalism; Caribbean.

Cosminsky S., (1975) "The Changing Food and Medical Beliefs and Practices in a Guatemalan Community", *Ecology of Food and Nutrition,* change; food beliefs; Central America; Guatemala.

Dirks R., (1987) *The Black Saturnalia,* University of Florida Presses, history; foodways; diet; nutrition; hunger; famine; social relations; slave society; Afro-Caribbean

Edelman M., (1987)" From Costa Rican Pasture to North American Hamburger", *IN Food and Evolution,* M Harris, E Ross (editors), Temple University Press.

Four Winds Food Specialists, (2002) *Population Profile: Puerto Ricans,* Fork, Fingers, and Chopsticks, food habits; Caribbean; Puerto Rico; North America.

Galler J, Ramsey F, Weiskopf-Bock S., (1998) "Infant Feeding Practices in Barbados Predict Later Growth" *The Journal of Nutrition,* infant nutrition; Caribbean; Barbados.

Greiner T, Latham M., (1981)" Factors Associated With Malnutrition in the Children of Western Jamaica", *Ecology of Food and Nutrition,* nutritional disease; children; Caribbean; Jamaica.

Handler JS, Aufderheide AC, Corruccini RS., (1986) "Lead Content and Poisoning in Barbados Slaves", *Social Science History,* history; slave diet and disease; lead poisoning; Caribbean; Barbados.

Hassig R., (1981) "The Famine of One Rabbit: Ecological Causes and Social Consequences of a Pre-columbian Calamity", *Journal of Anthropological Research.*

Jones AR., (1985) *Diet Change and Human Population at Indian Creek*, Antigua. American Antiquity, prehistory; Caribbean.

Kearney M., (1972) *The Winds of Ixtepeji*, New York, foodways; diet; food sharing; drinking patterns; Mexico; Zapotec.

McLeod J, Omawale., (1984) "Food Consumption and Poverty in Rural Jamaica" *Ecology of Food and Nutrition*, undernutrition; hunger; poverty; Caribbean; Jamaica.

Myers RA., (1984) "Island Carib Cannibalism", *Niewe West-indische Gids*, cannibalism; Caribbean; Island Carib.

Nietschmann B., (1974) "When the Turtle Collapses, the World Ends" *Natural History*, food use; ecology; Central America; Miskito Indians.

Ortiz de Montellano B. (1990) *Aztec Medicine, Health, and Nutrition*, prehistory; history; cannibalism; Mexico; Aztec.

Price R., (1991) "Subsistence on the Plantation Periphery: Crops, Cooking, and Labour among Eighteenth-century Suriname Maroons" *Slavery and Abolition: A Journal of Comparative Studies*, history; food habits; Caribbean; South America.

Tucker K, Sanjur D., (1988) "Maternal Employment and Child Nutrition in Panama" *Social Science and Medicine*, child nutrition; Central America; Panama.

Vargas LA, Casillas LE., (1992) "Diet and Foodways in Mexico City" *Ecology of Food and Nutrition*, diet; eating patterns; food preparation; nutrition; urban areas; Mexico.

Watts D., (1984) "Cycles of Famine in Islands of Plenty: The Case of the Colonial West Indies in the Pre-emancipation Period", *IN Famine As a Geographic Phenomenon*, B Currey, G Hugo (editors), famine; history; Caribbean.

INDEX